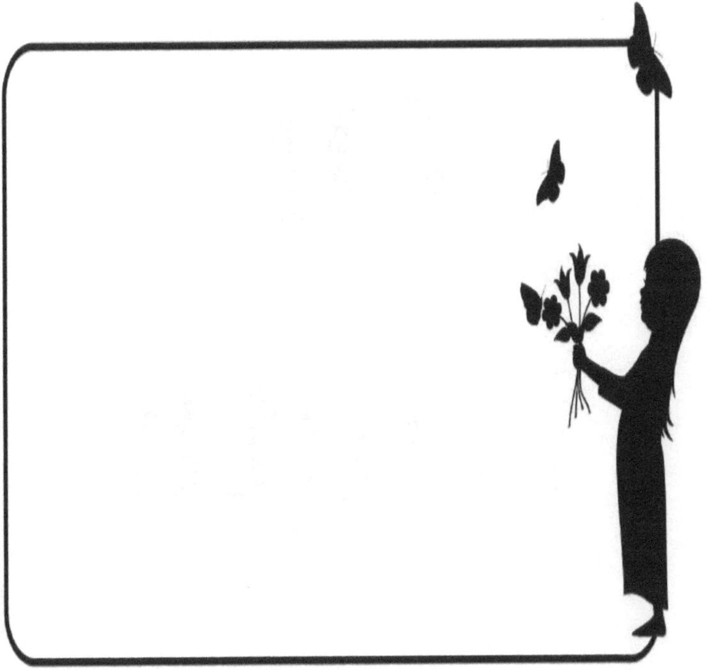

Secret Of Youth

Brian Obodeze

The issue of longevity is hardly taken into consideration until a certain "age of enlightenment". For most people, health consciousness begins in the middle ages when your body begins to experience less than satisfactory changes. The aging process differs from one person to the other and from one gender to the other. It is very unlikely that a person's health status can be defined by their age; rather, it is more to do with internal, external, and genetic factors. In this book, we explore these factors and sequences in a fun and in-depth way; excavating the more important and most trivial aspects of our being. Physical, mental, and emotional aspects of our lives are explored in detailed scenarios that allow near-accurate profiling, providing answers to the true secrets of youth.

Table of contents

Chapter 5. How the body works

- Cells
- Tissues
- Organs
- Systems
- Body metabolism
- Vital key terms: Telomerase, Dyschromia, Melanogenesis, Collagen synthesis

Chapter 6. Introduction to mental health

- Emotional health
- Physical health
- Correlation between physical health and mental health
- Aging and Midlife crisis
- How to handle the midlife crisis

Chapter 7. Empowering your body

- Diet
- Calorie requirements
- Hygiene: Haircare, Skincare, Colon care
- Natural remedies and combinations
- Lifestyle: Social life and activities, Sleep, Yoga, Workouts

- Career (how to reduce stress in the workplace)
- Deteriorating habits on mental health
- Natural remedies for mental health
- Cognitive-behavioral therapy
- How relationships can cause mental health problems
- The solution to relationship problems

Conclusion

Top 20 best websites for health tips

Chapter 1

Understanding your body

'How old are you?' – A common question that you or anyone would impulsively respond to without a second thought, especially if you were in your childhood and glorious teenage years. As you gradually depart from your twenties and thirties, you become a little more uneasy and calculated in your response. Perhaps as you answer, you're also paying attention to the looks on the face of the one who asks – do you see indifference? Do they seem impressed, surprised, or does their facial expression depict a downright 'what the F**K!'

Now don't get me wrong, aging is a beautiful thing but almost in everyone's subconscious mind, the mental countdown goes something like this:

15 years "Woo!"

20 years "Woo!"

25 years "Woo!"

30 years "Wait."

35 years "What's going on?"

40 years "Oh God!"

50 years "Please make it stop!"

60 years "I will give anything"

While it is an absolutely normal phenomenon and a bit of a disaster that we are all sliding into the big decline (old age) with the speed of a bowling ball, are there imminent signs that your body may be aging a little faster than you really are?

Since your mirror will not do more than throw a reflection of your image back at you without any further assessment, it might be fun to play a little investigative game. If we asked a dozen strangers to take a guess at our age and we took the average value out of their guesses, some of us may be in for a little surprise!

Yet, it isn't too late to arm yourself beforehand. You're about to be exposed to a lot of stuff you never knew about growing old and the very secrets of youth that many dermatologists and professional health consultants wouldn't tell you for free!

First, understand the process of aging. The human body can be likened to a company hiring new workers from time to time and implementing new policies for its smooth running and as the years go by, the company stops hiring. Workforce begins to drop drastically until the company is no longer as successful in carrying out operations as it used to be and then it packs up. This metaphor best describes the aging process of the human body.

Our bodies, while we're still young, reproduce billions of cells every day (about 242 billion daily for an adult and over 100 billion for a child). As we grow older, the body's ability to replicate cells decreases from time to time. So, on average an adult loses between 50 – 70 billion cells daily while a child loses 20 – 30 billion per day. Again, the body creates non-functional cells that interfere with the normal cellular activities – all these lead to a deterioration of the body functions and at this point, we are faced with old age and all its ugly caprices. This is just the first part of the aging process.

The second part encompasses the damaging of cells which leads to the shortening of DNA. When cells are undamaged or normal, they carry DNA fragments in their mitochondria compartments. As we grow older, the cells become damaged by free radicals and our DNA comes under attack, this leads to acceleration in programmed cell death – this is known as apoptosis.

It would be clearer to think of the aging process as a paper manufacturing company where tons of papers are produced on a daily basis with the available trees in the company's plantation.

Over time, there is a peak in the demand for papers in the market, the company's increased activities are damaging to the existence of the plantation. The plantation runs out of mature trees and it takes the company some time to plant new ones which would take years to grow back. What happens during the wait? The company runs out of resources and eventually, papers, and the company folds up. This is what happens to our bodies, the aging body finds it difficult to reproduce cells quickly enough to replace the dead ones. The most obvious way to observe this is through our skin; it simply thins out and loses luster.

The third part of the aging process disarms our body's own soldiers; natural antioxidants, weakening their defenses against free radical attacks that are harmful to our bodies. Little wonder why aging comes with an upsurge of illnesses and health disorders.

Aging, also known as senescence, can, therefore, be defined as the process of growing older. The process is usually genetically and environmentally controlled. It is a pile-up of several different changes in humans and these changes are typically physical, psychological and social. We will get to discuss these three factors later on.

There might be a nagging question at the back of your mind, like 'why?' Why does the above-mentioned company stop hiring and why do the trees take so long to grow back? Looking at these two questions, you would find that while one is environmentally controlled and is a result of human decisions, the second is a completely natural course; a combination of these two factors is what influences aging.

What makes you age?

The vigor of youth begins to slow down with time and this process is quite relative to various individuals. A young virile and energetic jock might begin to fade from "John Wick" to "John Weak" with absolutely no clue as to how to slow down this aging process. Is there something you should know about aging? Well, yes there is.

So, we do know that cells die; the real question is why and how? Cells die in several ways, some of which include lack of oxygen or too much heating, poisoning and infection but suicide is not one of the options many of us would likely consider. Well, cells actually do kill themselves too!

When cells die uncontrollably, it is likely to damage surrounding cells – this happens because they swell up and leak away. In conditions where they are in control of their death, it becomes a programmed cell death, this is known as apoptosis. Apoptosis is a much tidier process of mass cell death and humanly normal.

Apoptosis is required in human development, for instance during the early life cycle of a human being, the embryo is formed with webbed feet, it is this apoptosis that occurs in between the toes on the feet in order to separate them and ensure a normal formation of the body.

When apoptosis occurs, it is able to remove the contents of the dead cell spills so that it doesn't come in contact with surrounding cells and cause damage to them.

In order for us not to deviate, we are going to focus on why cells actually die. Every day, there are harmful molecules that attack your body; these usually come from what you consume and environmental factors. For instance, one of the worst culprits is glucose (a kind of sugar), another bigger culprit is the free radicals. Free radicals are by-products of energy produced. Glucose... (I think you should take a seat at this point).

Glucose

Glucose is an important source of energy and normally, your body breaks down carbohydrates to achieve glucose which, well, your brain actually needs. With age, there comes a problem with having glucose around because they stick to your proteins and create a cross-link which alters the proper functioning of your proteins. When cross-linking happens, it makes your blood vessels to harden. That's not all; it also damages your kidneys and nerves! These are some of the serious problems faced at old age.

What did they say free radicals are again?

Free radicals are molecules that can cause damage to the healthy cells of our body, causing us to age both internally and externally. Our bodies are vulnerable to attack from trillions of free radicals which are produced in our bodies through normal chemical reactions brought about by our daily activities. These activities include exposure to UV sun rays, pollution, stress, strenuous activities, smoking, and drinking.

It is good to note that smoking is a bigger culprit as each cigarette introduces trillions of free radicals into the lungs, this has spurred the warning on every tobacco pack or ad: *smokers are liable to die young* – this is because they age a lot quicker than non-smokers, besides the increasing possibility of lung cancer and other health disorders.

Internally, when our bodies are overexposed to free radicals they damage lipids, DNA and proteins and for that reason, our internal organs, including the brain, degenerate faster. Externally, it damages the cells especially those ones responsible for the suppleness and youthful elasticity of our skin. The older we grow, the more its effect on our skin becomes visible. In order to properly assess the indicators of aging on our skin, we observe wrinkles, pore size, evenness of color, UV spots and porphyrins.

The two culprits mentioned above both have the ability to destroy the fats, proteins, and DNA of which our cells are made. Note that the damages caused don't necessarily pose a problem of replacement when you are still young, but as you age, the reverse becomes the case.

How lifestyle impacts on aging (comparison between Mr. Riley and Mr. Sam)

Our pace of aging has a lot to do with our daily lifestyle. There are no limits to the way our lifestyle actually influences our tendencies to age quicker and the subsequent development of age-related health conditions. While aging cannot be completely deterred, scientists have proven through years of ardent researches that a certain lifestyle can slow the aging process and make you feel much younger. We are going to take a closer perspective of this by observing the difference in the lifestyle of Mr. Riley and that of Mr. Sam both in their late forties.

Mr. Riley's weekend:

Mr. Riley has had a hard day's work on a Friday and when he's back home it's time for some relaxation. First, he nibbles on his Fritos Corn chips and cheeseburger. He wishes that the weekend would last forever because he hates his job. He's grudging over his superiors who do not seem to understand why he gets to work late from commuting a straight route every morning. Since his work pays the bills, he keeps it anyway. The weekend obeys Mr. Riley, it's seemingly pretty long after all he hasn't been doing much, he's the typical couch potato.

Spanish la Liga keeps him glued to his seat as he enjoys the match with bottles after bottles of chilled beer. He's had too much to drink; he needs some food in his system. He passes by his push-up stand and stationary bike and approaches his fridge. He opens the big cold machine and shoves his hand through the mass of broccoli, and lettuce leaves, carrots and some other veggies and gropes for a can of spam with cheese and a loaf of bread cake. He enjoys a quick fix of his canned food and bread while sitting in front of his television. He gets so full he grabs a stick of cigarette from the pack and lights it. It's pretty cold that evening and several sticks of cigarette sound more 'warming' and exciting than sliding under his duvet for some sleep. He empties the cigarette pack.

At night Mr. Riley makes it a point of necessity not to miss out on his midnight movies, tomorrow's still weekend anyway. He sits on his couch with dark circles under his eyes screaming in awe as the car racer on TV crashes his automobile into another's.

In the morning, he wakes up on his couch realizing he had fallen asleep there. He gets up groggily, passes by the dusty treadmill and heads to the toilet for a poop. It wasn't until the last poop dropped into the bowl he suddenly thought *shit, the weekend's actually over and I'm late for work...again!*

He gets to the office pretty late, tired and grumpy, so grumpy he can't wait for another weekend to come by.

Twelve implications of Mr. Riley's lifestyle:

From the typical day-to-day of Mr. Riley's life, a few things were noted. As normal as his life may seem to a lot of people, there are underlying dangers; some of the components of his lifestyle are factors that contribute to aging faster. Here's what we observed:

1. Die-hard commuting
2. Junk food champion/ unhealthy dieting
3. Poor hydrating habits
4. Grudging
5. Couch potato
6. Alcohol
7. Smoking
8. No exercise
9. Poor sleeping
10. High consumption of processed foods
11. Poor social life
12. Lack of mental exercise

Unfortunately, Mr. Riley's day-to-day living is very similar to the lifestyle of billions of people around the world. This is why the World Health Organization (WHO) has come up with the fact that the pace of population aging around the world is facing a dramatic upsurge way higher than the past decades.

Not-so-fun fact: Out of roughly 150,000 people who die across the globe, about 2 out of 3 actually die from non-age-related causes.

Now, let's observe the life of Mr. Sam.

Mr. Sam's weekend:

Mr. Sam has had a tiring day at work, he's glad its Friday – the weekend gives him ample time for a whole lot of activities. He commutes on his way back because he had taken a walk to the office that morning; it was his golden rule. When he gets home, he takes a warm bath and eats some vegetable salad, fresh juice, and nuts. He likes nuts particularly; it made him really thirsty and makes him consume a lot of water. He liked to drink a lot of water even at his first waking at the early hours of the morning.

He takes a nap after eating, checks his mail later and watches his favorite TV program. Just after that, he decides to do a little evening exercise followed by yoga. He likes yoga because it gives him private time to meditate.

He finds time to visit his friends and relatives and catch up on their lives and share their deepest thoughts, fears, problems, and hopes. His evening is as vivacious as he had planned it. He gets home by 7:30 pm for dinner and afterward, he listens to relaxing music and goes to bed.

Saturday morning, he hits the gym for some exercise and weight lifting till he's all sweaty. He goes home takes a shower and fixes himself a breakfast of apple-cinnamon oats and salmon fish meal.

He cleans up his apartment later in the day, reads a book and catches up on a date that evening.

When he gets home he only eats apples and a couple of bananas and retires to bed. The following day, he tidies up his apartment and gets enough nap. The night before work, he goes through his mail, puts down plans for the week, and makes important notes of events and things to do at work. This exercise sets his mood for resumption tomorrow, he sleeps early and wakes up to a bright Monday morning with the spring in his steps and the weekly cycle goes on and on.

Twelve implications of Mr. Sam's lifestyle:

1. Strict rules on morning walks
2. Healthy dieting
3. Good hydrating habits
4. An active lifestyle
5. No grudging
6. Adequate daily exercises
7. Smoke-free
8. No alcohol

9. Adequate sleep
10. An active love life
11. Good social habits
12. Mental exercises

Verdict:

Mr. Sam's lifestyle is by far healthier than Mr. Riley's. His consumption of healthy, antioxidant fruits and veggies will help reduce the attack of free radicals in his system as well as keep his calorie intake minimal. He does not undermine the power of keeping his body hydrated and his early morning water therapy does more wonders than you can imagine to his body.

His highly active life full of both physical and mental exercise will help consistent blood circulation, the fitness of body muscles, repelling of excess fats as well as maintaining a sound mind. By reading and yoga practices he gets enough time to exercise his brain thereby keeping off most mental diseases that come around with aging, such as Alzheimer's disease, poor cognition, and memory loss.

So comparing the lifestyle of Mr. Riley with that of Mr. Sam we've decided to pick out the destructive habits noticed in Mr. Riley's life and emphasize the good points noticed in Mr. Sam's as a combination of these efforts would help anyone stay young and stall the process of aging successfully.

1. Keep away from cigarettes: smoking is the fastest way to lung cancer and heart disease, all of which can cut your life short. Keeping away from smoking and even second-hand smoking is a good way to keep away from its dangers.

2. Moderate alcohol intake – alcohol infuses your cells, inflames your liver and damages your genes when consumed frequently and in large quantities. The recommendation for alcohol intake is a glass of wine for women and not more than two glasses for men.

3. Restrict your calories in order to achieve a longer life. When you cut off excess pounds you put fewer burdens on your system.

4. Drink more water - The older we get, the more our bodies' water content decrease. Dehydration is a serious condition in adulthood and should be avoided. Drinking water in the early hours of the morning does a whole lot of things: it helps your body create new blood cells and muscle cells. It helps you lose excess weight and boosts your body's metabolism. It cleans your stomach, purifies your colon, helps your digestive system to function properly, helps remove toxins from the blood and helps the skin to glow. All these make you look years younger than you are. Four glasses of water or a liter daily is a perfect amount. You can begin with less and gradually work your way up.

5. Social life – socializing as you grow older boosts the quality of your life and can greatly improve your mental and

physical health. When you stay connected to your friends and loved ones you will benefit from their social support, which in turn will ward off stress, anxiety, depression and help your cognitive abilities. All these are likely to reduce the occurrence of some age-related diseases

Chapter 2

What happens when you age?

If you can pinch out one whole inch of skin on your forehead, then it's official, you're getting there. Getting to the point of your later life may not seem very pleasant for you because as the saying goes: time heals but it is a very bad beautician. So people are often two-faced about aging as some think it's only good because it is better than the next alternative.

Aging happens both internally and externally as we know. While the external changes are more obviously seen e.g. bodily features, the internal is usually felt. We would like to categorize the qualities that come about with aging into Physical, psychological and social changes for more clarity.

Physical changes

Physical changes that occur with aging can cause a lot of worries, especially for women, about physical attractiveness and desirability, job security and social status. Physical changes vary from person to person and this is a lot dependent on lifestyle and genetic factors as some people do not look as old as their age while some look a lot older. Some of the other changes that scream old age are as follows:

External physical changes

- Greying of the hair. The sudden appearance of a gray pube might just be God's way of saying "Alright, start wrapping things up." Your hair turns grey at around 50 years of age and you start losing some of your hairs, this is called pattern hair loss. This hair loss will usually affect 60% of men by age 50 and 40% of women the same age. The onset of hair thinning and greying usually goes from panic to use of medications and hair regrow products to a gradual acceptance of balding at later years.

🔲 Skin wrinkles – this usually happens because of photoaging and mostly affects areas usually exposed to sunlight e.g. the face. Your skin becomes drier and you sweat less. Due to the decrease of the skin's subcutaneous fat which is responsible for its good looks and supple texture, shrinking and wrinkles occur. Before you go suspecting that there's mass production of fake moisturizers in every cosmetic store, you should probably think of nature's course hitting hard at you.

🔲 More visible bones – since you store less fat beneath your skin, your skin becomes thinner and less elastic that's why. So as the body mass decreases, you look frailer and your bones tend to show through your skin. By the way, those bones may not hold you up as smartly as it used to and joints may feel the impact. It wouldn't be unusual if at some point you begin to ask "hey guys, remember when you could still refer to your knees as right and left instead of good and bad? Such good times!"

🔲 Features change – earlobes droop, chin sag, spine slightly arcs and you walk with a forward lean, etc. musculoskeletal changes and reduction of body composition continue to occur. Others include loss of bone mass in the face, thinner lips, sunken cheeks, and more projecting temples.

Internal physical changes

- ▢ Your heart slowers
- ▢ Your bones and muscles grow weaker
- ▢ Digestive system slowers (swallowing becomes a huge task for your esophagus)
- ▢ Your immune system weakens - remember what we said about free radicals attacking your system! At this point, you are more vulnerable to diseases.
- ▢ Your senses decline – poor eyesight, lower hearing, and lowered speech. This is usually the peak of cataract treatment, as well as glaucoma and macular dysfunction. There's more difficulty seeing in low lights. Colors are differently perceived so don't even try to guess the colors you see on that pretty rainbow up there!
- ▢ Your kidney and urinary tract is less efficient – they become smaller and develop decreased ability to remove waste
- ▢ Hormonal disorders - at this point female fertility issues caused by irregular cycles are most likely to occur before menopause consequently kicks in.

Gynecologist: After 28th when's your next period ma'am?

Ma'am: Sometimes again next year...God willing!

- Changes in the nervous system – the brain's ability to send signals and communicate to the rest of your body reduces. This is the reason for some neurological disorders at old age, e.g. Alzheimer's disease, Parkinson's disease, etc.
- Changes in body clock – you could experience one or more vagaries that you just can't point a finger on. For instance, you may begin to wonder why you're up at the same time in the midnight, just like yesterday and the day before…and the day before. In another scenario, you may not understand why your body needs to shut down at a particular time of the day or night, every day and you begin to recline into your shell more often, needless of a proper reason.

You: I can't hang out late on Friday night buddy

Buddy: Why not?

You: I'll be having a headache on Friday night

Psychological changes

- Cognitive ability declines
- Memory loss
- Inability to focus
- Reflexes slow down

Social changes

- Loneliness and social isolation
- Retirement
- Marital status and widowhood
- Typical daily activities
- Availability of caretakers

Aging between married couples

A relationship and marriage counselor takes her time out in figuring out recurrent patterns in the behaviors of her clients. She finds out one thing for sure, her female clients are in emotional distress over their husbands having affair(s), but that's not what she finds uncanny. She discovers that her clients have had a very smooth, romance-filled marriage up till the moment their husband's clock between the ages 40 – 50. It is surprising that most of them admit that once their men hit that age, they begin to sneak around and have hidden affairs with other women. So Ellen is all set to find out what usually happens to these men once they hit their forties. She notes down a few questions:

- Does a man's libido peak at 40-50 years?
- Does emotional attachment decline at that age?

- Does marriage matter less to a man when he's 40 years and above?

She intends to find out the answers to these questions by having a close-talk with her male clients about it. At the end of the sessions with her married male clients she gets the answers to the above questions:

- A man's libido does not necessarily peak at ages 40 – 50 years. In fact, a man may begin to experience a slow drop in libido followed by occasional erectile dysfunction which happens to 12% of men aged 40, 18% of men aged 50 – 59 years.

- Regarding emotional attachments in marriage, there may be a decline in marital satisfaction for both parties in the first fifteen years of marriage in many cases due to changes in identity, roles, and family pressures with the addition of children. However, the condition greatly improves along the line as children grow older and couple interests and values are reinforced. So in all, this does not mean there's significant emotional detachment.

- It's hard to scale how much one's marriage matters to an individual at a certain point in life amongst other spheres of life such as career and social lifestyles as this varies from person to person. The basics, however, remain the same:

emotional security, sexual satisfaction, companionship are for a good number of men, the basic expectations and purposes of marriage. In all, there is nothing that correlates men in their 40s and beyond to indifference or positivity of attitude towards marriage.

Ellen then carries out an interview with the same married male clients and asks them all the same questions and uncannily, they all said the same thing or similarly the same. Ah-ha! She says to herself as she figures out the obvious truth.

In as much as there are no hard rules to age differences between couples, studies in both western and non-western countries including within African have shown that women are socially inclined to be with men who are 5 - 10 years older than they are. The difference could be slightly lower than 5 years or slightly more than 10 years. So usually, when a man is in his 40s the wife would be anything between 30 – 35 years and when a man was in his 50s; his wife was likely between 40 – 45 years. At the age of 30 – 45 years, there are bodily changes that occur on these women which are slightly heightened when they have birthed a child or several children. Usually, these changes come as a combined result of the age factor and pregnancy-related changes which, in most cases, leave a permanent alteration in the body of the woman. Some of these changes are:

1. Increased body fats – while the accumulation of body fats may stop at around age 55 for men, it continues for women

up till about 65 years. The most common type is the belly fat. Women accumulate fats in their mid-region, arms, thighs and several other areas. This is the reason why exercises and dieting are things a woman at this age range must never overlook.

2. Changes in the breasts – menstruation alone brings about short-term changes in the breasts, making it fuller, for the duration of the period but pregnancy and childbirth magnify this effect. During pregnancy, the milk ducts grow in readiness to nurse a baby. After nursing, the breasts attempt to return to its former size but this isn't completely successful. However, it becomes less full and elastic; this results in a sagging of the breasts which is irreversible. Accumulating more fatty tissues around the breast area can however improve its outlook. The sagging intensifies at the onset of menopause due to the decline in estrogen hormone levels in the body.

3. The vagina after childbirth – there's been a subtle argument over this: does the vagina get back to its pre-pregnancy size? You bet not. "Almost" might be the right answer to that because it really does puts in some great

efforts. What do you expect when the size of a baby's head has passed through what used to be just finger-wide? Does he notice this? Maybe! Just try some kegel exercise to be on a safe side.

4. The skin – a woman's skin is taut until around 50 years of age and then it begins to grow thinner, drier and less elastic and wrinkles gradually become more visible. Fine lines may begin to appear as early as 30 – 35 years of age. This is worse if the woman has lifestyle habits like smoking, drinking alcohol and high daily exposure to harmful ultraviolet rays.

5. A decrease in libido – the sex drive of your early twenty may begin now to decline, this sometimes depends on how sexually active you are. Women with high sexual activity are likely to keep up with the trend even when the long arms of old age pull at them than their other female counterparts.

6. Post 35 mood swings – as the years go by, you are likely to encounter emotional changes on your way to the big forties and beyond. Call it a mid-life crisis or whatever, it might just come in the form of crankiness, stress and even depression – this can have an effect on your spouse and the entire family. You just may not know what's keeping your partner a few inches away from that expected romance.

7. Stretch marks – those worrisome ugly lines that show up from nowhere during pregnancy or after childbirth can often be a cause for worry. This usually occurs as a result of the weight gain and loss that happens before and after childbirth. If you are lucky enough, it will vanish, and if you aren't...now that's the problem we're talking about.

Age is nothing but numbers...agreed, but could you use that sunscreen on the table on your way out, please? You don't want to have more spots than a cheetah or more burns than muffins in the oven.

Look at all the above-listed changes, not one would cross a man's mind upon a falling star. If you think a combination of all the above isn't enough to keep your partner worried in the bar or in the arms of a mistress, I understand your plight but we are all full of imperfections!

Ellen advised her clients that a long-term marriage plays a great role in the lives of aging couples. Numerous studies have been conducted over the past 150 years and most suggested that marriage is actually good for the health and that there was a correlation between the two, a major survey involving 125,545 of adults in America found that married men are actually healthier than their unmarried, widowed and divorced counterparts. Scientists, after evaluating 3682 people over a period of 10 years found that marriage benefits the heart, it reduces social isolation, depression and even though it would not reduce the risk of cancer, it would affect the outcome. In general, married men had a 46% lower death rate than unmarried. Another study of 27,779 cancer patients revealed that patients in stable marriages had a better chance at survival than unmarried or separated ones. Similar survival tendencies were found in married men with prostate and bladder cancer. Other benefits include better retirement life, better cognitive abilities, reduced risk of Alzheimer's disease, and improved blood sugar levels, etc. while STDs in unmarried and widowed men were recorded to be a lot higher.

Ellen also advised couples to often look beyond the physical changes that happen, especially in a woman's body in her mid-life or after pregnancy and childbirth, reasons being that childbearing is beneficial results of a union. *"Look at it this way," she says "One of you had to do the job right? And natured bestowed it upon women, if these changes cannot be reversed with exercising and healthy diet courses, it shouldn't call for a big fuss since bodies and their responses differ."*

Now let me debunk something real quick. If you are wondering that if childbirth comes with all such dramatic changes then it's not too advantageous to the woman's body. Child adoption can solve it all right? Wrong. With all the thorns on roses, we still haven't lost the awareness that they are roses. Childbirth actually does come with some benefits many do not know! It has the ability to deter some of the illnesses associated with old age. Below are some **privileges** women who do not give birth tend to miss out on:

- Brain functionality – your brain works better after childbirth and this can be explained. During pregnancy and after childbirth, the brain expands in size in order to meet up with both mother and baby's needs. Neurobiologists explain that childbirth is a big stage in a woman's mental development and this spurs their work efficiency in rates much higher than in women who do not have kids.
- Reduced risks of Alzheimer's disease – scientists in Canada discovered that even after a baby has been delivered there were still deposits of the baby's cells in 68% of the women tested, this means that a physical connection has been created. These cells penetrate the placental boundaries are found in the brain of the women. The upside? Male cells in the brain of a woman reduce the chances of Alzheimer's disease.
- Active body and healing abilities – embryonic cells help women's wounds to heal faster and also heals and wards off serious diseases. Scientists discovered that the liver biopsy of a woman with hepatitis C began to self-heal, even after

she ceased treatment, because of her embryo. A great example of nature's miracle!

- Decreased risk of cancer – after childbirth it seems as though an anti-cancer switch has just been flicked on in the body of a woman. This includes ovary cancer and endometrium. As pregnancy progress to full term, the risks decrease the more and women who breastfeed their babies become less susceptible to breast cancer.

Are men excused from the prowling tentacles of old age as regards their bodies? You bet not! How their partners tend to handle it varies from one woman to another. Here are some of the physical changes that occur in men from 40 years and above:

- More lines and wrinkles
- Increased hair growth in unusual areas of the body e.g. ears, back, nose, etc.
- Your prostate grows more, at this point, it is time to get a frequent prostate examination to avoid Benign Prostatic Hyperplasia and urination issues
- Major hair loss on the head (balding), this will affect more than 53% of men between ages 40 – 49
- Belly fats, a signal that there needs to be a cut down on high calorie and fatty foods
- You become visibly shorter
- Graying of hairs
- Your penis size appears smaller and erections decline as testosterone level drops off

- Male fertility declines too

Chapter 3

The problem with aging

Before people turn old, watching old frail and women move across the road with walking sticks and the pace of a snail was something that seemed far-fetched, now as they come to terms with reality, they figure out that they should have prepared much better in their days of youth. How fast can the aging process be? Think of it as a roll of tissue paper, the nearer it gets to the end, the faster it becomes.

Old age actually comes with numerous issues, if you had a bad lifestyle, it would scold you in its own way like a nagging parent to a stubborn child. Sometimes it would pull you to the side, regulate you, ground you, and get you living just the way you ought to, many times it's just a thorn in your frail flesh. It interferes with your daily life as you begin to deal with the following issues:

1. Sensory changes: *"Do I smell vegetable salad or has little Danny pooped again?"* when you hear yourself say this, understand that your sense of smell has gone haywire. Other sensory changes include hearing loss, decreased visual acuity (presbyopia). Vestibular function declines so dizziness and falls frequently occur. *"yeah, I don't do alcohol anymore, I get the same effect just standing up fast"*

Your taste buds aren't exempted: *"More salt please...more...I mean more!"* Your salt detection has taken the day off...every day. Your taste bud for sweetness is usually unhampered but your bitter buds are exaggerated. So, wonder less why certain green vegetables are a nightmare.

2. A decline in muscle mass and strength – this already begins to happen to a lot of people after their fourth decade of life. *"Finally, I've stopped eating pickles. It's not that I can't open the jar though."* Significant loss of muscle mass and strength, known as sarcopenia, begins to happen fully at the age of 85. Sarcopenia is also caused by reduced hormone levels, severe inflammation, impaired muscle stem cell, and mitochondrial functions.

3. Immunosenescence – the immune system faces various attacks at old age. The body faces changes such as a decline in B cell function, decreased generation of T cells resulting to decreased natural immunity, at this point, the body may be too weak to fight off infections. This is the possible reason for the higher susceptibility of influenza infections and herpes in old people which has proven unresponsive to vaccines. This decreased inflammatory process is also the cause of slower healing of wounds in aged people. *"Another bruise? I guess time only heals in the afterlife!"*

4. Urological changes – an accumulation of bacteria may occur in the urinary bladder, this may be asymptomatic and occurs more in older women than in men. In fact, 50% of women stand the risk. Diseases in relation to this factor are not treatable with antibiotics as attempts may lead to bacterial resistance.

5. Slower walking speed and mobility disability – "why does everyone tell me to hurry up on a hike!" This often occurs as a result of aging and more so when there is an underlying disease. Slower walking speed falls, mobility

disability and risks of mortality do increase. On average, 1.1 m/s walking speed has been recorded for men within ages 85 – 89, while for women 0.8 m/s is the average speed. It is advised that aging people should partake in daily physical activities in order to improve their walking speed.

6. Disability in various activities of life – no wonder aged people need caregivers and have various facilities around the world to cater to their needs. This becomes necessary as their ability to bathe, dress, cook, use the toilet, and take medications, etc. declines. Studies have shown that 75% of people around the age of 85 have most or all of these disabilities, however, this number seems to slowly decline in the past few decades according to research.

7. Frailty – severe weight loss makes the aged weak, slow and easily exhausted. This leads to more falls, hospitalization and unsuccessful surgeries. This has called for nutritional recommendations and physical therapies for the aging as 35% of people in the age range of 85 – 89 are found to be frail.

8. Decreased cognition and dementia – *First you forget names, then you forget faces, then you forget to pull*

your zipper up then you forget to pull your zipper down. Memory loss increases as a result of impaired brain functionality and the processing speed of information equally declines. However, cognitive decline itself does not occur in totality as the brain fights to retain and process fractions of information. Aged people living with dementia live in decreased safety and increased dependence on caregiver supports and technologies that assist in their daily living.

9. Depression – No, this is not a usual symptom of aging, however, the other surrounding factors of aging can increase the tendency of depression especially those hospitalized or institutionalized as a result of disabilities. Another factor such as retirement/ lack of income and low quality of life also contributes. This is more prevalent in aged people of 70 – 85 years of age.

10. Social isolation – being wealthy and staying in a fulfilled marriage can extend an aged person's survivability. Social isolation, however, occurs because older people usually stay indoors with no much reason to be out there

except a doctor's visit and pressing needs. Those who completely live alone are more vulnerable.

11. Living arrangements – while some aged people appear to do better in their homes, some require institutional placement; this is usually decided upon by family members after an assessment of their preferences and safety of the aged one.

12. Adverse drug effect – this usually occurs due to polypharmacy. As older people face higher risks of disease, there is usually a high prevalence of polypharmacy among them. Polypharmacy is the use of 5 or more medications by one person. This increases the chance of drug-drug interactions and adverse drug effects.

13. End of life care – as an aged person approaches life's end, life-sustaining therapies such as mechanical ventilation, cardiopulmonary resuscitation, tube feeding, etc., are given some consideration. Death they say is inevitable, but you can cheat it off a few seconds, maybe days, weeks or months!

Diseases associated with aging

Diseases occur from time to time, but also they are age-specific in most cases. For instance, measles, mumps, and chickenpox are childhood associated diseases and are not expected to suffice in old age. So also we have old-age-related diseases. By popularity, these diseases include but are not limited to the following:

1. **Atherosclerosis** – this happens due to vascular remodeling, a diminished elasticity of the arteries and a buildup of plague – all these processes make the vasculature stiffen. This disease begins earlier in men than in women by 10 years difference.

Global Statistics of Atherosclerosis: This disease is the leading cause of vascular diseases all over the world. World Health Organization has estimated that 31% of all deaths worldwide are related to cardiovascular diseases. It is prevalent in 18% of young adults 20 years and above.

2. **Age-related Macular Degeneration (AMD)** – this disease affects the vision and can lead to blindness in one eye or both. AMD can be classified as either wet or dry. Wet AMD happens due to the blood vessels close to the retina which causes the Macula to swell. Dry AMD causes have not been properly established but it is believed to be partly as a result of the breakdown of some tissues and light-sensitive cells around the macula.

Global Statistics of Age-related Macular Degeneration (AMD): studies have proven that 5% of blindness all over the world occurs due to AMD. I96 million people will have AMD in 2020 according to research. The major causes are age, genetics and tobacco smoking.

3. **Alzheimer's disease** – As a person ages, the abnormal proteins are deposited in some parts of the brain and these deposits are neurotoxic and lead to cognitive degeneration. This is why people with Alzheimer's disease have poor cognitive abilities and memory loss.

Global Statistics of Alzheimer's disease: Alzheimer's disease is the most common type of dementia that happens with senescence. At least 50 million people all over the globe are living with this disease or some other form of dementia. Rate of increase in sufferers are meant to reach 182 million by 2050

4. **Benign prostatic hyperplasia (BPH)** – this disease occurs when there is an abnormal increase in the growth of the prostate gland which can block the bladder and affects a man's ability to pass urine. Studies have shown that 10% of men will have signs of this disease at the age of 40 and at the age of 86, over 90% of men are prone to having BPH. Reduced stream of urine, slow urinating, overactive bladder and inability for the bladder to completely get emptied during urination are all symptoms that are usually observed with this disease.

Global Statistics of Benign prostatic hyperplasia – one-third of men aged 50 years and above will be affected by this disease. It is 90% prevalent in men aged 85 years all over the world.

5. **Hypertension** – this disease contributes largely to atherosclerosis. It is associated with senescence and can even lead to mortality. Hypertension, especially the isolated systolic type is commonly found in people 60 – 80 years of age. Many blood pressure treatments aim to achieve goals of less than 140/90 mmHg in all older patients and less than 150/80 mmHg for non-frail elderly ones. The earlier intervention will prevent irreversible damage to the arteries and accelerated vascular aging.

Global Statistics of Hypertension – studies have shown that an estimate of 1.13 billion people all over the world suffer hypertension. Hypertension is a major cause of untimely death and two-third of sufferers live in low and middle-income countries. As of 2015 1 out 4 men had hypertension while 1 out of 5 women had it.

6. **Cancer** – this is another disease that leads to mortality. The ability for a sufferer to respond to cancer treatments

actually depends on the physical status rather than age. Detection at an early stage and aggressive treatment are highly advised in order to prolong the life of a sufferer. While normal body cells grow and divide and stop growing when they should, at the occurrence of cancer, what happens is that cells are abnormal grow out of control and spread really quickly, they also do not die when they ought to.

Global Statistics of Cancer – according to the World Health Organization cancer has caused 9.6 million deaths in the year 2018 and over 18 million new cases were recorded. It has been observed that 1 out of 5 men and 1 out of 6 women develop this disease during their lifetime.

7. **Diabetes Mellitus** – Many times this particular disease is linked with peripheral neuropathy and peripheral artery disease which contributes to diabetic foot ulcers and subsequently leads to amputation. It is also associated with cardiovascular diseases which all occur at old age. 6% of all diabetic patients develop foot ulcers yearly and about 0.5% of them are amputated.

Global Statistics of Diabetes Mellitus – According to the world health organization, diabetes is more prevalent in low and middle-income countries and has recorded 422 million cases in 2014 from its previous record of 108 million in 1980.

8. **Osteoporosis** – As you age, your bone density begins to decrease. This disease is most common with people aged 85 and is normally associated with an increased rate of fractured bones. It is advised that women over the age of 65 get a bone screening while the occurrence is suspected to affect men aged 85. It is believed that calcium and vitamin D supplements can help prevent its occurrence, however, this is yet unproven.

Global Statistics of Osteoporosis – Studies have shown that this disease is bound to affect about 200 million women all over the globe once they've clocked 60 years of age and above. It affects 75 million people in the USA, Japan, and Europe.

9. **Arthritis** – Rheumatic Arthritis (RA) can occur at any given age but is more prevalent among people aged 30 – 50 years. However, when it begins at the age of 60 and 65, it is referred to as elderly-onset Rheumatic Arthritis. Older men and women get RA at almost the same rate but in younger people, women are more likely to develop RA. It usually happens in specific joints such as your toes and fingers and its other symptoms include fever, muscle pain (myalgia), anemia and weight loss. In order to minimize its chances of occurrence, physical activities such as exercises and other therapies are highly recommended.

Global Statistics of Arthritis – World Health Organization has estimated that 9.6% of men and 18% of women aged 60 years and above are suffering from osteoarthritis. While 25% of this population will be completely disabled by the disease, 80% of them will have limitations in mobility.

10. **Cataracts** – cataracts come in the form of a cloudy area in the eye lens, this is very common with old age. Its other symptoms include a blurred vision, fading colors, double vision, sensitivity to light and difficulty seeing at night. This eye disease can be corrected through surgery only. Studies have shown that half of all Americans around 80 years of age or older, have cataracts or have undergone the surgical treatment of it.

Global Statistics of cataracts – According to the World Health Organization, there are 18 million cataract sufferers who are bilaterally blind. This illness remains the leading cause of blindness all over the globe.

Obesity and aging

I can't wear my white jeans, it's out of shape, it's tight on the waist but loose in the legs, I'll work on my white jeans…and on my red and on my blue…black…yellow. They're all out of shape, I'm not!

Hey, stop right there. Before you begin to worry about your clothes, you should put your new size on the top of the worry list. While weight loss is a common factor during the aging process from 65years and above, the reverse is the case for some. Usually, older people begin to lose body mass as it is only normal that the body is able to cope when it doesn't have to deal with more body mass than it can handle at a certain age. However, obesity has been observed in some people as they head towards their 60s, this commonly includes the accumulation of visceral fats. This can be a worrisome factor as aging already has its other issues and being overweight is not one of the things you want to battle with at a time when exercising is most difficult. When people become overweight in their old age, they become vulnerable to the chronic diseases that happen to obese people such as

- Type 2 Diabetes
- Hyperlipidemia
- Hypertension
- Atherosclerosis
- Obstructive sleep apnea
- Liver dysfunction

While these associated diseases can occur in obese people in all age groups, it has more dire consequences in elderly people due to their immunosenescence. Obesity at old age is not only highly linked with chronic ill-health, but it also paves the way to a disability, poor quality of life and functional decline.

What causes obesity among the elderly?

Your energy intake vs. your energy expenditure is the major determinant of your body mass. When your calorie consumption exceeds your calorie expenditure, then there comes a buildup of body mass. When you age, your consumption level does not necessarily decline and there could be a decrease in the expenditure especially from 50 to 65 years of age – this is what causes obesity at old age. Other causes are:

- Genetic factors
- Environmental and sociological factors (physical activities and lifestyle)
- Other illnesses (e.g. hyperthyroidism, polycystic ovary syndrome)arthritis, Cushing's syndrome and depression
- Drugs (e.g. anti-depressants and steroids)

Don't be afraid to spend an extra buck to fight off obesity such as devoted dieting, health supplements, frequent medical checkups, slimming herbal beverages and exercise equipment, it will save you the cost of medical bills in the future at the onslaught of chronic ailments. Developing the habit of visiting the gym frequently is one of the best natural ways to ward of obesity as you age.

"Dear old age, you've shackled out joints tight, folded our once tight tummy in multiple steps, thank you very much. Now pay for our gym sessions."

- *Anonymous Obese*

Why do women live longer than men?

Old age is considered a better option than the next alternative, no matter how much people detest the effects of old age, many would still want to live long. You would have probably heard of the old myth that women outlive men by a greater percentage right? Except that this really isn't really a myth or old wives' tales. Statistics have proven countless times that this is true and the reason isn't much of a surprise.

In the United States, several pieces of research have revealed that men have 60% higher death rates than women and in 40% of the death rates in men, there's a link to some health conditions brought about by their own lifestyle. Yes, lifestyle...again!

There's been a noticeably higher rate of arteriosclerotic heart disease, lung cancer, emphysema, etc. and other diseases related to smoking. A higher percentage of smokers were found among men than in women, so was cirrhosis of the liver caused by heavy alcohol intake. The other death causes are linked to aggressive activities, being adventurous, taking on hazardous jobs that equally place them at the forefront of mortality than their female counterparts. Some other sort of behaviors that are more accepted for men by society than for women, this includes the handling of guns and other weapons, engaging in dangerous games such as automobile racing. We observe all these without ruling out the occurrences of unprecedented accidents and suicides.

Again, some things are wrongly viewed as feminine and only exclusive to females, these things include body and skin care, dieting and maintaining certain body standards. Other self-soothing actions like shedding emotional tears are also wrongly considered feminine and are hardly acceptable for masculine standards set by men. Whereas shedding tears has great health benefits, it releases oxytocin and increases your sense of wellbeing. It greatly relieves stress, fights bacteria, improves vision, releases toxins and promotes good sleep. All these benefits can be freely enjoyed by anyone, regardless of gender.

Chapter 4

Aging gracefully and aging wastefully

An ad caught my attention – In a lonely desert, a middle-aged Chinese woman was wailing with her dying lover in her arms. She wished and prayed that somehow her lover would survive as they were distant from life and he was badly wounded and near death. At that moment, out of a little whirlwind came a genie. The moment she saw the genie she had a feeling of triumph, she knew instantly that something miraculous was going to take place.

"Make just one wish and I will make it come true," said the genie. Her fingers trembled anxiously as she looked at her lover with eyes filled with tears of hope. "You mean any wish and you would make it come true?" she asked the genie.

"Yes, any wish."

She breathed out and shut her eyes for a few seconds and then she opened them, smiled up at the genie and passionately exclaimed through her breath "Give me a youthful skin like that of sixteen years old!"

It wasn't hard to see the look of confusion and slight disappointment in the eyes of the poor genie! But he granted the wish anyway.

How much are women willing to give up on beauty and secrets to a youthful look? Tens? Hundreds? Thousands of dollars? Even a dying wish upon a genie?

Anti-aging products are the order of the day because they sell off in tons, to say the least. Let's take a look at how much money goes into the cosmetics industry all over the world.

If you were to go to Sephora.com – a Paris based multinational chain of skincare and beauty products or the likes of Sephora and type "anti-aging", you would be lost in a sea of thousands of shopping options and millions of products. In the year 2021, anti-aging products alone would have consumed a whopping $330 billion globally in products such as creams, masks, oils, serums, and tools. The figure is highly feasible due to the fact that anti-aging creams are way more expensive than your normal moisturizers and for obvious reasons; they claim to do a lot more and many of them contain some specialized ingredients. For example, the popular La Prairie Skin Caviar cream alone gulps a staggering $197,880 yearly and this is just for a minuscule cream that would barely last three weeks. This example is one of the hundreds of thousands out there!

Some of the natural ingredients used in these anti-aging products include coenzyme Q10(C oQ10), salicylic acid, Cova B Trox, sepilift DPHP, nutria ceramide, vitamins, emollients and tripeptide among others. Some products are anti-oxidant based while some are probiotic.

Technological anti-aging treatments are increasingly becoming on popular demand, some of them includes:

- Stem cell technology
- Anti-aging wearables
- UV detecting patch
- Dermo patch
- Mitochondria for youthful skin
- Anti-wrinkle serum
- Lip plumpers
- Laser skin resurfacing
- Telomerase activator

⯈   Sun protection factor (SPF) in skincare products

A lot of global players in the cosmetics industry reel in more money from anti-aging products, such brands include Avon, Chanel, Christian Dior, Ella Bache, Estee Lauder, Clinique, Johnson & Johnson, Neutrogena, Revlon, Pfizer, Elizabeth Arden, Unilever, etc.

So, we have a whopping figure on the expenditures surrounding the anti-aging cosmetic industry, but are anti-aging options strictly restricted to money? Here's a little story below to answer this question.

Sally and Deborah

Mrs. Sally lived near Mrs. Deborah and that was all they shared in common or so they thought. Sally was unmarried and lived alone while Deborah was married to a US marine who was often away on duty. Mrs. Sally was however scared that she would not be able to continue living in such a highbrow area as the house rent was becoming too much for her to afford. Also, living next to Mrs. Deborah, the rich lady made it more obvious that she was living a below-average lifestyle and this impacted negatively on her self-esteem.

Sally would watch the pizza delivery man go to and from Deborah's house with a smile which suggests generous tipping. She would watch her order of energy drinks and expensive vodka (her favorites) being delivered too. She would sit back drearily and eat her own budget-friendly dish of beans, peas and lentils and an apple for dessert. She made a mental comparison of the kinds of food she eats and that which Deborah eats. She's had heard numerous times that healthy foods were more expensive than unhealthy foods and for the obvious reasons, but she had a way of picked healthy choices without breaking the bank. Also, she knew that food-related health issues such as diabetes, heart diseases, and cancer aren't usually included in the cost of your unhealthy junk when you buy them, so even though they are referred to as "Cheap", how cheap can they really be on the long run? Some kinds of beverages were a big no for Sally, for instance, she didn't have to take energy drinks, they were caffeinated and once hooked she knew she would not be able to constantly afford it. Besides that, energy drinks had the tendencies of increasing the blood pressure and chances of heart diseases. So sally made home-made natural fruit juices, they were cheaper anyway. She asked herself if it was a healthy comparison she was doing or was she secretly envious of the things that her neighbor Deborah could afford.

Every single day, she always knew when Mrs. Deborah had just arrived. She knew the sound of her car – an expensive SUV. She went everywhere with it, it was as though she could not imagine why would she own flints of cars and begin to stroll down to the groceries, mart or wherever she wanted to go. Sally wished so hard that she was in Deborah's shoes.

Deborah held parties at her apartment too. One day she came knocking at Mrs. Sally's door

"You're invited to my house party this evening. Young ladies like you light up a party."

Sally felt flattered, it seemed much like an older woman acknowledging her. Deborah was much older than she was anyway,

"...but please Sally...please put on a pretty dress"

Mrs. Sally warmly accepted the invite feeling a little anxious about the dress part; she had to put on her favorite gown to look at least proper. The party would be filled with the rich folks so she needn't look out of place.

 As soon as she was ushered in through the door of Mrs. Deborah's house it was a wonderful sight. The people were colorfully dressed. She narrows her eyes through the fogginess of cigarette smokers to find Deborah seated beautifully in a lovely black dress smoking and drinking with her friends. She spends only a few minutes at the party, she didn't like the smell of cigarettes in the air.

Years go by and it was only once that Deborah knocks at sally's place. *A casual visit? Another party invitation?* Mrs. Sally wondered.

As Deborah came in and took a seat, it was obvious she had only come to check up on her neighbor and then her eyes caught a familiar old school badge somewhere on a wall frame.

I know that school, that's the school I attended "Metropolitan girls high school"

"You attended the same school as I did?" Sally exclaimed and then the familiarity in Deborah's face came vividly. How could she have missed that? She thought. Then Deborah reminds her of the exact set and they happened to be classmates although Deborah had changed school at some point and left much earlier. They share a hearty hug. "How could we not have known this a long time ago?" Deborah said and then Deborah's face begins to change, she suddenly looked curious. "How could you have been the same set as me and not sets below? Sally. You are very much younger."

"What do you mean?

I mean…how old are you Sally?"

"I'm thirty-nine"

Deborah thought that Sally was being silly, people reduce their ages and not otherwise.

"Liar. You know it's uncool to try to make me feel we're also age mates, you really don't have to shoot up your age"

"That's my age Deborah," Sally said with a face full of smiles.

She paused looking at Mrs. Sally, she was looking 27! And compared to her, her face and skin were still aglow. She had no fine lines on her face. She was slim and fit too.

"Are you really 39, Deborah?" Mrs. Sally asked. It wasn't hard to see the looks of shock on her face as she waited for an answer. Deborah obviously looked 52! At that point, all the envy she felt for Deborah vanished - she had lines and slight wrinkles, she was slightly plump too. Thanks to all that pizza and alcohol she consumes almost on a daily. As Deborah sat there, she decided on what to do, she was going to buy back her youth! The answer to it all was in her pocket! Sally had something she didn't have and she had something Sally didn't have ...money. That was the secret to youth, she thought, with a smug look on her face...*Money*. She had no idea how wrong she was.

At Mrs. Deborah's office, her colleagues are having a rather strange conversation about her.

"Have you seen Debbie lately, she's a fine wine. The older she gets the younger she looks"

"Debbie? Last I saw her before my leave she looked pretty much like my granny. She's all wrinkled up"

"I think I saw her yesterday, she's looking like a sweet sixteen"

"Shhh guys...she's on Botox, get it?"

Let's take a break on Sally and Deborah

Our stand on Botox

Botox is a drug made from botulinum toxin type A, this toxin is usually gotten from the bacterium Clostridium botulinum. This drug is the most popular cosmetic treatment and reportedly gulps over 6 billion dollars every year.

Why do people use Botox?

Apart from its use for bladder and bowels condition treatment, migraines, excessive sweating, and muscular disorders, it has been found to have a counter-aging effect. As a cosmetic treatment, it is usually injected into the body and when this is done, it blocks out signals from your nerves to your muscles, thereby preventing the muscle in target from contracting. This is a method believed to improve the appearance of fine lines and skin wrinkles. It is currently considered 'celebrities' best friend' as it is commonly used among them. As a matter of fact, an increasing number of men have it injected into their scrotum to give it a better appearance than a saggy one. Lines, known as crow's feet that appear at the sides of your eyes when you smile and frown lines are usually reduced with Botox injections.

Is Botox the new anti-aging elixir?

For many, this method has been safe and effective since it is injected in small amounts, however, this should be done by a qualified medical professional who would be able to administer the correct amount of Botox in the right area. However, long-term efficacy is highly limited and lasts for 3 – 6 months. This will make one dependent on regular injections every six months. This is the very downside, you have to go for sessions several times in one year and it seems as though once you get a Botox shot you can't stop, you dare not stop. You don't want to go from beauty to beast in one blink of an eye. Yes, if you discontinue your wrinkles will return, the muscles in the treated area will start to function normally as was supposed to and this will return the aging process! This method of maintaining a youthful look is not only temporary for each treatment but may be out of the reach for the poor to the average person as the average Botox session costs 150 pounds – 350 pounds per session. NHS would only cover Botox treatments for certain ailments and conditions but would not cover for the purpose of cosmetic application. The price depends on how much Botox is used at each session. Its cost also depends on where you go to get the treatment and which areas you are treating. While making up your mind on where to go for treatment with the knowledge of this price range, bear in mind that 'cheap' has every chance to turn out unimpressive.

Also, while it may have no prolonged side effects some of its common side effects include:

- Numbness
- Redness of area injected
- Mild pain
- Headache
- Flu-like malaise
- Mild nausea
- Bleeding
- Blurred vision
- Double vision
- Fatigue
- Dry mouth
- Swelling
- rashes

Some rare side effects include temporary droopiness of facial features like eyelids or eyebrows, weakness, difficulty in swallowing and speaking, troubled breathing. Prolonged use may also lead to your body becoming resistant to the treatment…oops! Now that's leaving you in the middle of nowhere.

Sally and Deborah continued…

The next time Sally sees Deborah she looks different and Sally figures the right word for the difference *"Younger!" No way! It was like magic!* It would be rather awkward to mention a word about it to Deborah after the awkwardness of their last conversation. She, however, admired Deborah's new looks secretly.

Five months later Deborah was on the phone with her husband (who was talking about coming back home soon) when she casually faced the mirror as she often did with as she was obsessed with her new looks and she gets a hint of surprise. Her voice begins to waver on the phone as she felt uncomfortable with her mirror image – she was beginning to notice her wrinkles again, even the crow's feet at the sides of her eyes were quite obvious. She rushes her husband off the phone and hangs up. She needed a visit to the dermatologist who gave her Botox treatments. As she drove she wondered how many people had seen her, how many people had noticed the changes! As she sat waiting for her turn she flips open the latest edition of Vogue magazine, her idol, Angela Simmons had graced the front page. Angela was an ever-young celebrity with sultry looks. She read part of the interview where Angela admitted *"Yes, I've done several plastic surgeries to enhance my looks. I'm proud of it too."*

Deborah slammed the magazine shut as an idea came to her head; she could end her visits to the doctor for Botox treatments in just one simple plastic surgery. She wouldn't bother to get a Botox treatment, there was no point sitting here waiting for her turn, she's got a better option. *I don't intend to do facelifts upon facelifts till my ears meet – It would be moderate, it would be just once and for all,* she promised herself. She was wrong, again. That was the beginning of her journey into plastic surgery and then several readjustments, which were still…err…surgeries!

Let's take a pause on Sally and Deborah

Our stand on plastic surgeries

When plastic surgery was incepted, it was majorly for medical use; restoring and reconstructing the human body. It was commonly used in caring for soldiers that were facially disfigured during the First World War. Now, the majority of use cases for plastic surgeries are cosmetic. We can also term it aesthetic surgery as it is majorly an inclusion of facial and body enhancements.

Cosmetic or aesthetic surgery is performed on normal body parts in order to improve its appearance and eliminate the signs of aging. Research has shown that in 2014, about 16 million cosmetic surgery procedures were carried out in the US alone and the total number has doubled up since the last century and 92% of these cosmetic surgeries were performed on women. The most common types were liposuction, breast enhancement, eyelid surgery, breast reduction, abdominoplasty, rhinoplasty (nose job), facelift, filler injections (collagen, fats and hyaluronic acid) 81% of these procedures were done on Caucasians. Cosmetic surgery has become popular in all parts of the world regardless of region and race, thereby rising 115% from 2000 to 2015.

Aesthetic surgery has been popularized by celebrities and media influence has played a role in endorsing these counter-aging techniques in subtle ways. But we do know that plastic surgeries are more complex than people actually think. First, patients of aesthetic surgeries battle with the disorder that comes along with it – the obsessive concern that one gets over his/her appearance after a surgical adjustment of the face or body parts. It is as though over half of the patients are often not pleased with the results and go back for subsequent adjustments. This becomes a somewhat plastic surgery obsession which is best described as Body Dysmorphic Disorder (BDD) - a condition that makes the sufferer preoccupied with their perceived bodily or facial defects and often manifests along with anxiety or depression. All these surgical redos come without a second thought that there is a limit to what the human can undergo.

Potential causes of BDD are filter apps like Snapchat and face tune. Snapchat dysmorphia makes patients request for surgeries in order to look like their photo-filtered version. BDD can lead to gross dissatisfaction, insecurity, and low self-esteem and subsequently suicide. Not to mention that many do not endorse plastic surgery as a solution to anti-aging for obvious reasons like complications, risks, and reversals. All surgeries are risk-bound, some of the risks encountered with surgery include:

- hematoma
- infection
- damage of nerve
- implant failure
- scarring
- rupture
- organ damage

Some surgeries necessitate future adjustments or reversal, for instance, a breast implant for augmentation will need to be removed after 10 years.

Sally and Deborah continued...

Deborah's cosmetic surgery was a success. The wrinkles were worked on; she got a facelift too and touched up the eyelids. She had spent a lot of money on it so it definitely looked worth it. But then again, she wanted the very best, she returned to the doctor for small touches on the rhinoplasty and face muscles. She stood in front of the mirror every day and saw beneath the beauty, all the little imperfections that could still be readjusted. Her visit to the doctor became equally as frequent as that of the botox treatment; the only difference was that this treatment was a lot more critical. Money bought her whatever she wanted whether they were the right or wrong things.

Her neighbor Sally had seen the improvement; she had noticed immediately that there was something about the sudden extra youthfulness and beauty in Deborah's look. Sally had been so observant that she noticed after years that her lips were getting slightly puffy and tight, her eyes were unnaturally bright, and there was something about her that was uncomfortable to look at. The effect came clearer as months went by, till it became really difficult for the neighborhood to set eyes on Deborah. She quit her job and got freelance work from home and it appeared as though she avoided been seen. She got paranoid whenever her bell rang.

One day, the bell rang and it was her long-awaited husband who had returned. She was really excited as she gave him a hearty hug, however, she couldn't discern the worrisome looks on his face. A week after Deborah's husband go back, his behavior had changed and he filed for divorce saying he was unable to connect with her as he used to as she had greatly changed physically. That night after Deborah had cried immensely to the news, she stood in front of the mirror with a few years old pictures of her and there in the mirror lies the answer to the sudden outturn of things. She had thrown her money on the wrong things; truly Sally her neighbor lived a simple life and didn't need to buy her own downfall, it became more and more difficult to believe that they were of the same age even though she didn't have the money to do whatever she wanted, she was able to take good care of herself. There are simple rules to youth and these do not really cost a lot, spending on the wrong things such as toxic foods, drinks, and plastic surgeries just to reverse the effects of aging will lead to what we should be permitted to call *the Deborah effect*.

Here are cheap ways to slow aging.

1. Water – it is very important to always hydrate. Drink enough fluids like water and natural juices daily.

2. Proper skincare – vital skincare tips include avoiding a really hot bath and over-washing your skin so as to retain its natural moisture. Also, use a good basic moisturizer for your skin (This mustn't be expensive). Cleanse the skin gently and keep away from harsh products.

3. Appropriate use of Sugar – sugar is best taken off of the dining table; it is best left in the bathroom. In many ways, using sugar outside your skin might just be a lot more beneficial than consuming it. Use it to exfoliate your skin by mixing with olive oil and scrubbing your skin so as to unclog your pores so that your skin can be better penetrated by the products you use.

4. Keep sugar intake moderate – Limit sugar intake so as to reduce the stress of having your body break down carbohydrate which could raise your insulin levels. A rise in insulin leads to inflammation which in turn produces enzymes that break down elastin and collagen and the end product is a saggy skin full of wrinkles.

5. Android-agers syndrome – sometimes, just put that phone down. Try as much as you can to avoid looking at screens a lot as it creates dark circles under your eyes unsuspectingly.

6. Use sunscreen – protect your skin from repetitive exposure to harmful UV rays.

7. Quit smoking – sometimes it's quite easy to tell a smoker from a non-smoker. The signs are usually obvious, dry chapped skin and lips and yellowed teeth. To have a reversed effect, stay away from the next stick of cigarette.

8. Drink less alcohol – alcohol dehydrates the skin and allows it age faster.

9. Eat healthily – there are lots of natural food options that are just a dollar or below. While craving your lean meat and fish meals, also concentrate on cheaper and equally beneficial options like grains, lentils, fruits, etc.

10. Reduce stress and get enough sleep – this includes mental and emotional stress. Sleep produces melatonin which is the body's antioxidant responsible for skin cell repair.

11. Exercise daily – this aids blood circulation and helps your while system working actively.

The Cleopatra way

Thousands of years ago, we didn't have those bank-breaking cosmetic creams and serums, expensive face masks and Botox treatment, the great queen of Egypt Cleopatra, known for her ageless beauty, made use of her kitchen foods and spices to achieve flawless skin. DIY skincare can be fast, easy, healthy and cheap! Here are some of those natural skincare tips that would do just what those expensive over the counter anti-aging products would for less.

- Avocado facial scrub for vitamin B

- Exfoliate with brown sugar and yogurt
- Tea tree oil for cleansing and antibacterial
- Oatmeal in hot water for soothing the skin
- Mashed strawberry for a brighter skin
- Yogurt and coconut oil for great moisturizing
- Lemon for cleansing and toning effects

Sometimes the best things in life are free...well, almost free.

Chapter 5

How the body works

When you look at a single person head to toe, there is certainly so much that goes on behind the scene that you do not see. Every human is able to sleep, wake, get up, poop, eat go to work or school and back, etc. and the cycle goes on and on. This smooth running of days, nights, weeks, months and years make it difficult to really imagine the activities behind the scene (inside a human body). Now let me take you on an interesting tour of the human body.

Just like they say, the human body can be compared to a machine with different functional parts and each part has its own unique function, yet all the parts work in unison to perform one primary function. The different parts of the human body are at various levels and the initial level begins with the cell.

We can, therefore, categorize parts of the human body according to its level of complexity in the following order: Cells, tissues, organs, systems

1. Cells – the cell is the basic part of the human body and an average adult has trillions of cells in the body. It is the basic unit of life as it is present in all living things and is important for their survival through its vital processes. There are various kinds of cells performing specialized functions according to the department of the body in which they exist. We have
   - blood cells
   - surface skin cells
   - bone cells
   - columnar epithelial and goblet cell
   - cardiac muscle cells
   - skeletal muscle cells
   - neuron
   - Smooth muscle cells

All these cells are uniquely created to function in the specific part of the body they are built for. For instance, the nerve cells carry electrical messages to other cells, it is shaped with long projections that helps it carry out this unique duty, while muscle cells have numerous mitochondria that help to supply the energy required for the movements of the body.

2. Tissues – This level in the organization of the human body comes right after cells in the human body. The tissue is a cluster of cells that are linked together and perform like functions. We have four kinds of tissues in the human body namely: Epithelial, nervous, muscle and connective tissues.

    i.   Epithelial tissue – this kind of tissue is comprised of cells that cover the inner and outer surfaces of the body like the skin and the lining of the respiratory tract. The epithelial tissue is protective of the body's surface and organs inside the body.

    ii. Nervous tissues – this type of tissue is made up of nerve cells otherwise known as neurons that carry electrical messages. The neurons make up the brain and send brain signals to other parts of the body.

iii. Muscle tissue – this type of tissue is built with the natural abilities to contract, elongate and shorten, this makes body movements possible.
iv. Connective tissues – it is comprised of cells that make up the skeletal structure of the body such as the cartilage and bone.

3. Organs – the organs come after tissues in the human body. It is more complex than tissues in the sense that it is a structure of two or more tissues combined to perform one function. Examples of organs are the brain, heart, liver, skin, kidney, and lungs. The organs in the human body play a specific and vital function. For instance, the heart transports oxygen, hormones, and nutrients to the cells in the body while expunging waste and carbon dioxide from it. The skin is a protective cover of the body which also fights off infections and controls body temperature. The brain collects, transfers and processes information and signal. Kidney removes extra water, salts, and waste products from the body and controls the ph. balance of salt and water. The lungs carry air through the body so that gas exchange can take place between the blood and cells.

4. Systems – This is a group of organs that work to fulfill a complex function. We have several systems that make up the human body; this includes the skeletal system which gives structure to the body and internal organs. We also have the muscular system which enables bodily movements.

The digestive system breaks down food and absorbs nutrients in the body. The respiratory system takes in oxygen and releases waste in gas form. The nervous system controls thoughts, sensation, movement and other minor activities of the body. The circulatory system carries oxygen, substances, and nutrients through the body and removes waste.

Body metabolism

It would be incomplete to talk about aging and all the insufficiencies that occur in the body at that phase of life without talking about one of the most popular factors - Our NAD is a lot important to us. No, it wasn't a typo, I don't mean DNA (which is also very important). I mean NAD+! Let's find out what these really are.

NAD+ or nicotinamide adenine dinucleotide is a coenzyme that exists in all living cells. The presence of NAD aids the normal processes in living things. However, NAD+ levels are one of the things that reduce with age.

The NAD+ plays two major roles in the human body: it serves as a key factor in metabolism by turning nutrients to energy and it also helps by serving as a molecule that assists the proteins that regulate biological activities in humans. These two processes regulate oxidative stress in us and maintain the strength and health of our DNA and regulate circadian rhythms. Everything perfectly goes well concerning our NAD+ until we begin to age and why? We simply do not have an endless supply of NAD+, as a matter of fact, the older we get the lesser they become.

PARPS or Poly (ADP-ribose) polymerases and sirtuins are both groups of proteins in the human body but which cannot function without the NAD+. Sirtuins are termed by scientists as "the longevity genes" and its role of extending the life of cells is completely dependent on the activation of NAD+. That is in fact how important the NAD+ is to humans.

NAD+ has been proven to improve and restore mitochondrial functions in humans. Since the levels of NAD+ in a human's body could make or break the important processes in the body and NAD+ are typically gotten through the foods that are made up of amino acids, scientists are trying to produce an NAD+ supplement and they figured that giving regular doses of NAD+ precursor could greatly increase the levels of NAD+ in humans by 40%. So people who are aware of NAD+ would always likely watch out for supplements that boost the NAD+ levels while shopping for counter-aging supplements and other body boosters.

Some vital key terms you should know

- Telomerase (Its role in aging, tumors, and cancer) – telomerase is one of the natural combatants of aging in the body. It is an enzyme which tries to prevent telomeres (specialized repetitive DNA sequences and proteins in our chromosomes) from wearing down too much. As cell division occurs on and on, the body runs out of adequate telomerase which is meant to maintain the length of the telomeres and so the telomeres shorten and the cells grow old.

The two-faced telomerase:

The shortening of telomere and lack of telomerase has a tumor-suppressing mechanism since telomere leads to cellular aging and a stop in growth; this leads to the acceleration of the aging process but on the other hand, prevents cancer!

- Dyschromia – a number of things can happen to the skin of an aging person, this includes color pigmentation of the skin, as well as the nails and hair. Dyschromia is an alteration of the color of the skin or nails. While hyperchromic refers to hyperpigmentation, and hypochromic, hypopigmentation, dyschromia is an embodiment of the two conditions.

- Melanogenesis – this is the process by which melanin (a dark pigmentation) is produced. Melanin can be eumelanin (black to brown) or pheomelanin (yellow to reddish-brown). It is the ratio of eumelanin to pheomelanin that determines the color of the hair, eyes, and skin. Melanogenesis, which is the production of melanin, depends on both genetics and biochemistry. These discolorations among other causes could occur as a process of skin aging. Its excessive and anomalous distribution leads to skin spots and blotches and can sometimes occur as a result of menopause in women.

- Collagen synthesis – A lot of women are often familiar with the word 'Collagen' this is because it is written in many skin products. Collagen is the skin structural protein that makes up 75% of our skin. Collagen is comprised of 3 protein chains joined together. 33% of the protein in the body is collagen and protein structure has high tensile strength. Collagen is a strong element for the beauty of the human skin. It is the strength of the collagen that gives the skin that healthy, plump, smooth looks of youth. Collagen is created by fibroblasts. Fibroblasts are cells found in the dermis that create elastin (another structural protein responsible for the skin's ability to snap back) and glucosaminoglycans (GAG - The element that keeps the skin hydrated.) Fibroblasts, once naturally signaled by the body begin to reproduce collagen. The biological process of collagen production is altered with age, lifestyle and other environmental factors such as harmful UV rays.

Chapter 6

Introduction to mental health, emotional health, and physical health

Mental health is the existence of our emotional, social and psychological well-being. The way we behave, respond to stress, think, act and feel depends on the level of our mental health. Mental health problems may occur in a person due to the following factors.

- Family history
- Life experiences

- Biological factors

Duncan is just an ordinary man like every other man. He has behavioral patterns that are peculiar to him. Well, since no two individuals are alike, it might be just normal that he has his atypical idiosyncrasies or is it? Let's analyze Duncan:

Sometimes he gets forgetful, to say the least. He goes to the office in the morning, he greets the people in the other department and when he gets to the door of his own unit, he figures out that he forgot the keys at home. He drops his bag and quickly takes a cab home. On getting to his house door he realizes that his house key is inside the bag which he had just dropped at the office, he had left it right in front of his locked office door. He sighs, rushes down the road to get a cab back to the office to get his bag, his shirt soaked in sweat. He takes his house key from the bag and goes home. He opens his house door and checks on the table where he left his office key and the table is empty. He stands right there and begins to laugh till tears came to his eyes – his hands had slipped into his pocket trouser and the key was right there the whole bloody time! He had slipped the keys into his pocket earlier before he left the house and had forgotten he did. He looks into his wallet, he's cash strapped so he wouldn't be able to take another cab. He treks back to work to report late humming the song 'dark times' by Ed Sheeran in his mind to stop himself from screaming as he walked back to a 30km far office, set to face his waiting boss over his lateness. Phew! Apart from this, a few other things do occur in Duncan's life, for instance

- He hears voices in his head

- He feels numb sometimes (it's as though nothing really matters sometimes)
- He's usually secluded
- He barely sleeps
- He fights a lot with people
- He experiences serious constant mood swings which affect his relationships
- Sometimes he feels so hopeless that he wants to harm himself or others who stare at him as though they could read his mind.

Ok, now here's what…Duncan has a problem – a mental health problem. Mental health is the absence of mental disorders. World Health Organization would emphasize that Mental health isn't only limited to an absence of mental disorder but the state of wellbeing of an individual in which he could function productively regardless of day-to-day stress. Here are some common mental disorder types:

1. anxiety disorder – this has several branches such as panic disorder, phobias, obsessive-compulsive disorder (OCD) and post-traumatic stress disorder (PTSD)

2. mood disorder – this includes branches such as bipolar disorder, major depression, persistent depressive disorder, seasonal affective disorder (SAD)
3. Schizophrenia – the big schizo is the king of mental disorders. It is a complex disorder of which research is yet to determine if it is a single disorder or a group of fragmented illnesses.

Duncan's girlfriend who was almost getting fed up had set him up on a date with a counselor where he was given professional mental analysis and advice. He also advised Duncan on numerous ways to connect with people, get enough sleep, think positively and improve on his coping skills.

Emotional health

Emotional health is often used interchangeably with mental health but they are not the same. Having good emotional health means that you have the ability to manage the ups and downs of life. It is, in fact, a great skill. It comprises of a feeling of contentment, resilience, and self-awareness. A positive person is likely to be in control of his or her emotions and will, therefore, have a healthy emotional state.

Good emotional health equals the following:

- Better relationships
- Flexibility to stress
- More dynamism

- Better self-esteem

Here are ways in which you can improve on your emotional health as you grow:

- Practice emotional regulating activities that can easily slide you out of upsetting moments, such as meditating, seeing a therapist, writing and listening to cool music.
- Exercise – taking a walk or engaging in some form of exercise nourishes not only your physical state but your emotional state.
- Connect more with family and friends
- Get enough sleep – this eliminates stress and makes you less vulnerable to anxiety and other negative emotional states.

Physical health

Physical health encompasses the condition of your body, from physical fitness to being void of diseases. Your overall wellbeing is impacted by certain factors such as lifestyle, environment, nutrition and diet, physical activities, human biology, and healthcare service. Assessing your physical health involves checking the following things:

- Bodyweight and body mass index (BMI)

- Blood pressure
- Blood glucose
- Cholesterol level
- Reflex tests
- Flexibility
- Muscular strength
- Body composition(body fat percentage)
- Endurance tests

Correlation between physical health and mental health

Physical health as we know it is quite different from mental health of course but they do often go hand in hand. In many cases, if physical health gets really poor it could leave one prone to developing mental health problems, so also poor mental health has every tendency to lead to physical health problems. Here are instances of how poor mental health can negatively affect physical health:

Studies have shown that people with some significant level of mental distress are likely to die from cancer by 32% than their counterparts with optimal mental health. Also, depression has been known to increase the risk of coronary heart disease.

Schizophrenia has also been associated with a higher risk of developing heart disease and a much higher risk of death resulting from respiratory diseases. One of the main reasons could be that people with mental health problems are less likely to get the healthcare services that they should and may likely not go for common routine checks like weight, cholesterol levels, blood pressure and glucose levels, and so would not be able to detect from the onset, the symptoms of any physical health conditions. They may also not be easily offered help towards lifestyle changes involving diet, cigarette and alcohol intake.

Aging and Midlife crisis

The term midlife crisis may have been overused even for false purposes such as after a slight disappointment or depression that follows after certain expectations have not been fulfilled in one's life but it is better to get a clear meaning of it. No, it's not that feeling when you as an upcoming artist have just completed your first demo and after watching the next Grammy awards you fall into midlife crisis - you weren't nominated for the demo! Midlife crisis is a transition of identity and insecurity in middle-aged people (45-64 years of age) in the consciousness of their growing age, which is mainly psychological and brought about by events in their life, and shortcomings of their accomplishments in life. The feelings which follow midlife crisis are typically remorse, depression, anxiety after an evaluation of their life. They get caught in the phrase "If I could turn back the hands of time" because they desire youthfulness once again and changes in their life.

Meanwhile, critics argue that midlife crisis is a combination of different stressors in life which add up to become a crisis and this is a result of the multiple roles they play as spouses, parents, employees, children and so on. It is strongly believed that it is triggered by aging in combination with problems and regrets that occur as a result of

- Physical changes associated with aging
- Career setback
- Spousal relationship (or lack thereof)
- Maturing children (or lack thereof)
- Aging or dead parents
- Discontentment in economic, health or social status

Midlife crisis is experienced by men and women differently, for instance, a man may experience a midlife crisis due to work-related matters or wealth and material acquisition. Some men experiencing a midlife crisis in the western world may typically desire the purchase of a luxury item such as an exotic car or the intimacy of a younger woman. For women, a midlife crisis may typically be triggered by evaluations of their roles in life and physical changes associated with aging. Some women experiencing a midlife crisis in the western world may typically desire some sort of cosmetic surgery procedures to enhance their looks and slower the process of aging. For men, midlife crises last about 3 – 10 years, while for women, it lasts for 2 – 5 years.

How to handle the midlife crisis

Regular exercises and maintaining a nutritious diet in the long term can help to boost one's physical and mental health as you journey towards middle age and further. Setting your goals earlier in life, planning towards it, making wise decisions, as well as significant changes earlier in life, can help spur the growth of one's career and economic status and prevent the occurrence of stagnation and subsequent regrets that follow a midlife crisis.

It is also important for one to focus on the flipside - turn the onset of midlife crisis to a positive phase by looking at it positively rather than negatively. You can do this by seeing this self-evaluation phase as a time for self-realization and personal growth.

Chapter 7

Empowering your body

If you have gotten to this part of the book then at this point I'd like to give you some congrats ahead. You are keen about knowing the very secrets of youth and you are about to have them right away! First, understand that empowering your body encompasses every aspect of your wellbeing. It also entails bridging the gap between your physical and mental health in ways that would not only prepare you to age gracefully but most importantly, slower the aging process 100%. These aspects of body empowerment involve diet, hygiene, natural remedies, lifestyle, workouts, career, mental health, and relationships.

Diet

Not everything is fit for the consumption of all and dieters are aware. While looking for its long term benefits, a person may decide to pick a specific type of dieting that best suits him/her. Let me introduce you to the different kinds of diets around the world.

1. Paleo diet – this type of dieting eliminates all intake of sugar, processed foods, and grains. The idea is to minimize the number of carbohydrates and glucose in the body in such a way that your body is left with no option but to make use of the fats in your body for energy. A typical paleo diet consists of fish, chicken, vegetables, nuts, fruits, oils, potatoes, eggs, and grass-fed meat.

2. Vegan diet – this kind of diet typically eliminates the consumption of meat and other animal products. This diet helps in the reduction of saturated fats and cholesterol. On the long term, the vegan diet minimizes the chances of obesity, high blood pressure, and coronary heart disease.

3. The blood type diet – this kind of diet matches people with particular blood types to their specific dietary needs for optimum health. For instance, people with type o blood are required to eat lots of high protein meals and if seeking to lose weight, they are recommended to eat more of spinach, seafood, broccoli and stay away from dairy products. While blood type A is recommended to avoid eat and eat mainly soy, vegetables and seafood to maintain a healthy weight. These dietary recommendations and restrictions differ across blood types.

4. The south beach diet – this focuses on controlling the insulin levels of the body by completely avoiding certain carbohydrates. It involves the selection of carbs, lean protein, and healthy fats generally.

5. The Mediterranean diet – this type of diet focuses on plant food and fresh fruits. It is a vegetable-based diet that eliminates too much meat intake in order to aid weight loss and controlled sugar levels. In addition to vegetables, it supports whole grains, fruits, and herbs.

6. Raw food diet – this kind of diet promotes the consumption of uncooked and unprocessed foods. It also eliminates the consumption of foods that have been pasteurized or produced with additives or synthetics.

This greatly reduces the carcinogens in one's diet as well as risks of inflammation while boosting energy levels in the body.

7. The ketogenic diet – emphasizes the reduction of carbohydrate intake which allows the body to burn fat, rather than carbohydrate as fuel and produce ketones through a process called ketosis. The foods required for healthy fats in this type of diet are avocados, seeds, oily fish, coconuts and olive oil.

8. Vegetarian diet – this type of diet is classified into subtypes: Lacto-vegetarian, fruitarian-vegetarian, lacto-ovo-vegetarian, Ovo-vegetarian, living food diet vegetarian, pescovegetarian and semi-vegetarian. The majority of vegetarians are Lacto-ovo-vegetarians, this means that apart from dairy, eggs, and honey, they do not eat animal-based foods. They typically have less body weight, suffer fewer diseases and have tendencies to live longer than meat consumers.

Balanced diet

A balanced diet is that which supplies your body with required nutrients from the six classes of food in order for your body to properly function. For instance, a combination of the following foods will give you the correct nutrition for a balanced diet: Fresh vegetables, fresh fruits, legumes, whole grains, nuts, lean proteins. This will supply you with the calories you need for daily living. Typically, growing children, pregnant women and those involved in high-energy activities require enough calories through a balanced diet.

Calories requirement

An average person is required to consume 2,000 calories daily in order to maintain their body weight but this requirement, however, depends on factors such as age, gender, and level of physical activity. Older adults and those who do heavy exercises require more calories than others and men require more calories than women. Here is an example of daily calories requirements presented by the United States Department of Agriculture (USDA).

Person	Age range	Calorie requirement
Children	2 – 8 years	1000 – 1400
Girls	9 – 13 years	1400 – 1600
Boys	9 – 13 years	1600 – 2000
Active women	14 – 30 years	2400
Sedentary women	14 – 30 years	1800 – 2000

Active men	14 – 30 years	2800 – 3000
Sedentary men	14 – 30 years	2000 – 2600
Active men and women	Over 30 years	2000 – 3000
ntary men and women	30 years	– 2400

The following most consumed foods in the US according to USDA contain 'empty calories' – cookies, bacon, sausages, cheese, cakes, energy drinks, doughnuts, ice cream, pizza, sports drink, and soda.

Hygiene

When we say hygiene, we refer to clean living habits that maintain our good health. Personal hygiene is those things we do to care for our bodies to keep them clean. The fact is that ignoring our personal hygiene results in an accumulation of germs, dirt, bodily secretion and food residue which can be detrimental to our health. Worse still, we contact diseases and infections through poor personal hygiene. In 2016, research showed that diarrheal diseases, tuberculosis, and lower respiratory disease have been listed in the top 10 causes of death; all 3 are commonly and easily spread through poor hygiene. Here are common ways to observe good personal hygiene:

1. Washing your hands - our hands encounter so much on a daily basis like touching, of surfaces, eating foods, shaking people, working and playing, etc. so they are prone to getting in contact with germs. Common infections such as colds, cough, flu, gastroenteritis, etc. are easily passed through unwashed hands. Washing your hands often with water and liquid hand wash after a toilet visit, coughing, sneezing, being in contact with animals or a sick person or before eating or carrying a baby is a great way to maintain good personal hygiene and keep illnesses at bay.

2. Dental care/ oral hygiene – this is important in order to stay clear of gum disease, tooth decay, bad breath, and oral infections. The best way to observe good dental care is to brush twice a day; morning and before bedtime, floss daily, change your toothbrush regularly, chew sugar-free gum and keep your mouth hydrated with water more often.

3. Bathing – this is obviously important in order to smell nice and avoid infections. Bathe every morning and

before bedtime. Bathe more frequently during hotter days to prevent an accumulation of bacteria.

4. Wash clothes regularly – never wear clothes you've worn before. Wash them after each wear so as to remove dirt and germs. This is important so as to smell good and keep germs at bay.

5. Clean cooking conditions – the kitchen is a home to bacteria breeding from leftover foods or raw foods. It can contaminate surface areas, water, and edible items in the kitchen. It is important to make sure the kitchen is always cleaned up and unwanted foods and dirt should be gotten rid of. Dishes, kitchen utensils, and tabletops should be kept clean and dry always. Use clean water and wash hands before cooking each meal.

6. Travelers' hygiene – no matter how much in a hurry you are to make that trip, always prepare for unforeseen circumstances while traveling. First, avoid contaminated water or foods that may cause diarrhea. Carry a hand sanitizer for use after visiting public places.

7. **Haircare** – so many things can cause damage to our hair if not avoided. Having healthy hair often comes as a result of good hair care practices. Here are some tips for healthy hair:

- o Wash your hair regularly but don't over-wash
- o Wash with cool water instead of hot
- o Use sulfate- and silicon-free hair products
- o Condition your hair after shampooing every week
- o Wash your hairbrush frequently
- o Allow your hair to air-dry
- o After washing, moisturize with natural oils such as olive oil, coconut oil, mustard oil, peppermint oil, and almond oil.
- o Don't change your hair color too often
- o Avoid using harsh chemicals
- o Eat healthy foods such as

8. **Skincare** – Good health is often obvious from the looks of our skin. If we take proper care of it, we can delay the natural process of aging and avoid having skin issues. Here's how:

- o Avoid too much sun exposure. Harmful sun exposure leads to premature wrinkles, age spots, and susceptibility to skin cancer. It is best to use a sunscreen with an SPF of 15 in order to protect yourself from harmful sun rays.

- Seek shade to avoid the sun especially during its intense hours, usually from 10 am - 4 am and wear skin-covering clothes,
- Avoid smoking. It makes the skin dehydrated and damages the collagen and elastin meant to give your skin a healthy glow.
- Eat healthy e.g. Lots of vegetables, fruits, lean protein, and whole grain
- Manage stress - stress can increase your skin sensitivity and lead to a break out of acne and other skin issues.
- Limit bath time. Do not over wash skin.do not use hot water
- Avoid harsh soaps and moisturize the skin daily with natural moisturizers.

9. **Colon care** – the colon is part of the body's digestive tract. It is often referred to as the large intestine or large bowel. The colon is something like the 'cleanup' guys in the human body. It plays the function of cleaning out the broken down food from the body. Food absorbed through the small intestine moves into the colon and is further broken down by the bacteria in the colon. The colon then prepares this broken down food to be released from the body. This vital process of the body requires a healthy colon to perform properly. Eating some kinds of food helps the process required of the

colon and also cleanses it. Here is some useful colon-cleansing diet to take daily:

1. Broccoli
2. Dark leafy greens
3. Raspberries
4. Milk
5. Oatmeal

These foods are high in calcium, fiber and vitamin D and these are highly useful for a healthy digestive system. These foods are to be eaten one at a time and not at once in order to avoid diarrhea or constipation. Other tips for maintaining a healthy colon include:

1. Eating high fiber foods
2. Drinking lots of water for hydration
3. Avoiding too much red meat and processed foods which have been found to increase susceptibility to colon cancer
4. Take probiotics for diversification of healthy bacteria in your colon

Natural remedies and combinations

Using natural herbs may be considered safe and beneficial to health, it is, however, best to consult with your healthcare provider before taking them especially if you are on certain medications. The top 10 following herbs are popular for their effectiveness and high health benefits:

1. Chamomile (flower) – this flower is considered a 'cure-all' by many. It has wound-healing qualities and reduces inflammation and swelling. It is also used as anxiolytic and sedative for relaxation and curing anxiety.
2. Echinacea (leaf, stalk, root) – this is typically used to cure flu, common colds and infections. It also has wound-healing abilities. Prolonged use can, however, affect the body's immune system so it should be used in moderation. Also, people allergic to daisy plants will likely react to Echinacea.
3. Ginger (root) – ginger is commonly used to treat nausea and motion sickness, especially during pregnancy. Its reported side effects include bloating, gas and heartburn.
4. Feverfew (leaf) – it is used to treat fevers, arthritis and prevent migraines. Its side effects include mouth and digestive irritation.
5. Garlic (cloves, root) – this is used to lower cholesterol levels and blood pressure. It is also known for its antimicrobial effects. Researchers are studying the role of garlic in the prevention of cancer. Large amounts of garlic should not be consumed right before a surgery as it may affect clotting.

6. Gingko (leaf) – the Gingko extract is used to treat asthma, tinnitus, bronchitis, and fatigue. It is also good for the improvement of one's memory and prevention of dementia and other disorders of the brain. The Gingko leaves alone should be used as its seed may contain toxins.

7. Ginseng (root) – this is also known as a 'cure-all' and as an aphrodisiac. It's generally considered safe for providing vitality but is not good for consumption in people with diabetes. Its side effects include high blood pressure and tachycardia.

8. Milk thistle (fruit) – this is used in treating high cholesterol and liver problems. It is also used to control cell growth in cancer among numerous other illnesses.

9. Saint John's wort (flower, leaf) – this herb is mainly used as an anti-depressant.

10. Valerian root – this herb is used to manage anxiety and sleeplessness as it is known to aid better sleep. It is also used as flavoring in root beer and some other foods.

Below is a table for some fruit combinations with various health functions.

Fruit combination	Function
Cherry + pineapple + blueberry	Anti-inflammatory
Grapefruit + kiwi + strawberry	Immune-booster
Fig + red grape + pomegranate	Antioxidant
Goji berry + watermelon + lemon	Detoxifying
Blackberry + papaya + cantaloupe	Skin beautifying
Banana + avocado + apple	Energizing

<u>Lifestyle</u>

Staying physically active in your autumn years may serve but without any form of social activity, you may still not enjoy that quality life that you desire. Maintaining relationships and building connections with others will also contribute immensely to your overall wellbeing. Staying socially active comes with benefits such as:

      i.   Maintaining good emotional and physical health

      ii.   Increasing cognitive abilities

      iii.   Quality sleep

      iv.   Better immune system

      v.   Increased longevity

As you gradually transit towards old age, the following social activities are highly recommended in order to enjoy a quality lifestyle:

1. Join a club or group - especially pertaining to your area of interest e.g. Golfing, reading, arts.

2. Reach out to family regularly - spending time with family members brings the feeling of warmth and security while keeping loneliness at bay.
3. Become a volunteer – volunteering within your local community will grant you a feeling of importance and accomplishment.
4. Join a senior fitness center – Here is where you can meet your peers and keep fit together.
5. Enjoy lifelong learning – join an adult education center where you can continually learn new things and broaden your horizons.
6. Try new technologies – do not shy away from modern gadgets, also embrace new and better ways of connecting with friends via social media platforms like Skype and other newer platforms.
7. Pick up a part-time job – whether you need this is not, going back to work will keep your brain and mind stimulated. It would help you associate with people on more intellectual levels and as a bonus, you will have extra money to serve you for the rainy days.

Sleep

As a part of your daily life never undermine the power of getting enough sleep as you age. Adequate sleep helps you maintain optimal wellbeing among other things, it enables the body to rest, repair and get ready for the following day. People benefit from adequate sleep in the following ways:

i.   Better productivity
ii.   Lessened risk of excessive weight gain
iii.   Greater athletic performance
iv.   Better regulation of calories
v.   Better response to emotional stimuli
vi.   Lesser susceptibility to heart disease
vii.   Prevents depression
viii.   Lower risk of inflammation
ix.   Boosts the immune system

Here is the breakdown of sleep recommendation for every person

Person	Age	Sleep hours
Newborns	0 – 3 months	14 – 17 hours
Infants	4 – 12 months	12 – 16 hours
Toddlers	1 – 2 years	11 – 14 hours
Preschool	3 – 5 years	10 – 13 hours
School-age	6 – 12 years	9 – 12 hours
Teen	13 – 18 years	8 – 10 hours
Adult	18 – 60 years	7+ hours
Adult	61 – 64 years	7 – 9 hours
Adult	65+ years	7 – 8 hours

Other than sleep, the practice of yoga has loads of health benefits as well. It exercises both the body and mind. Since human beings are physically, mentally and spiritually inclined, yoga exercises balance all three. Here are the main benefits of yoga:

- It helps in managing stress and anxiety
- It relaxes the mind and body
- It increases muscle strength and flexibility
- It activates the parasympathetic nervous system
- It promotes self-healing
- It enhances better focus and concentration
- It improves breathing and promotes peace of mind

Yoga

Yoga is one of the best things to do in your alone time. Having some alone time is very important as it can help you focus on yourself, rest and sleep. Most importantly, making out time to be alone could help you to do some meditation and self-evaluation. It is also the moment when you can read a good book to better your self and acquire some extra knowledge.

<u>Workouts</u>

Exercises are generally recommended for a healthier life but in order to turn back the clock, anti-aging exercises are the specific recommendation. For a sedentary person, muscle mass peaks in their 20s and begin to decline from then on. Exercises are beneficial for the following reasons:

- It increases energy levels
- It improves muscle strength
- It helps maintain a healthy weight
- It helps the heart
- It enhances brain function
- It boosts the immune system
- It reduces the risk of degenerative bone disease
- It reduces the risk of cancer
- It aids better sleep
- It enhances a sense of wellbeing
- It wards off depression and certain other mental illnesses
- It reduces the effects of aging

Resistance training among others is very vital as it focuses on the major muscle groups. Men and women required different kinds of exercise to bring the best out of their physical health and fitness. Here are some favorable exercises for women.

1. Squatting with dumbbells
2. Brisk walks
3. Swimming

4. Balance training – try shifting your weight from one leg to the other and try to balance on one leg at a time
5. Posture exercise – opposite arms and legs raise works on your back and core. An upright stretch helps to straighten the spine when repeatedly done.
6. Static pectoral stretch and calf stretch. Stretching at least twice a week, holding each stretch from 30- 60 seconds at least can be very helpful.
7. Press-ups and step-ups
8. Planks.

Best exercises for men's fitness include the following:

1. Squats
2. Lunges
3. Cardio
4. Yoga
5. Planks
6. Bodyweight resistance
7. Functional training

Most exercises for men are typically designed to work on their biceps, chest, core, quad, shoulders, back, triceps, glutes, hamstrings and calves. Here are the specific exercises that work on the mentioned body parts:

- Biceps, chest, back, and triceps – do the dumbbell incline curl by lying down on an incline bench and hold dumbbells over the chest. Lower the dumbbells to the sides of your chest with palms facing in do repeatedly.
- Core and shoulders – do the half kneeling rotational cable chop by attaching a rope to a cable station. Kneel on your right knee and rotate as you pull the rope past your right hip, this would greatly improve on your stability.
- Quads and calves – with your heels elevated, hold up a barbell across the front of your shoulders and squat repeatedly.
- Hamstrings – do the barbell straight-leg deadlift by holding a barbell and letting it hang at arm's length. Bend your knees slightly, push your hips back and lower your torso till its almost parallel to the ground. Repeat 10 times.

Career (how to reduce stress in the workplace)

Many employees deal with stress in the workplace, in fact, work has been identified as the major cause of stress in the US. This has also become a worldwide epidemic according to the World Health Organization as employees reportedly battle with the workload, job insecurity, and personnel problems. However, there are some strategies that can help to reduce stress in the workplace and help employees stay healthy while on that job. These strategies include:

1. Workplace exercise – mild exercise is a great stress reliever, so taking walks during lunch break help to ease the mind. Also, a subsidized gym membership will serve as a great workplace bonus and help workers relieve stress and maintain their health of mind and body.
2. Engage in social activity – employees who socialize with each other tend to make their work appear easier
3. Go to a quiet place to recline – whenever the stress accumulates, cool off at some quiet place. A coffee break at work can help relieve those stressful work hours.
4. Have a full massage session during the weekends. Massage unknots your muscles and reduces stress in the body.

As the employer, you have the capacity to relieve stress for your workers in order to improve work output in the following ways:

i. Recognize worker efforts. Small moves like complimenting your employees give them a boost and enhance their workplace positivity in the midst of stress. A simple 'thank you' card is definitely a booster.

ii. Revamping the office environment and making it work-friendly. Use soothing colors on the wall such as cool blue, mint green, etc. and having plants and flowers create a psychological stress-relieving effect.

iii. Quality coffee and a serving of healthy snacks can help put stress on hold for a while.

iv. Allow remote working and flexible work hours if possible.

Mental health deteriorating habits

To acknowledge the medicine for mental health, we need to familiarize ourselves with those little triggers of mental health problems. There are simple habits that impact negatively on our mental health and may gradually lead to serious mental health problems such as anxiety and depression if left unattended. Below are some of these simple but bad habits and most of us would be guilty of one or more of them.

1. Slouching: your physical posture and the way you walk tell a lot about your moods most times. Having more peps in your step will give you a psychological mood boost than slouching those shoulders and hunching. Now roll back your shoulders and lift up your chin. There you have it.

2. You take too many pictures: snapping everything alter the way you enjoy and remember those awesome

moments, so keep that on a minimal and enjoy yourself more instead.

3. Lack of exercise: are we overemphasizing this? No. Exercise of any form is one of the best mental health boosters.

4. Procrastination: whether you are anxious over tasks or scared of failure. Procrastination is worse off, especially for the sake of your mental health. Jump on it now.

5. Taking life too seriously: laughter is medicine. It is great for anxiety and depression. Laugh over jokes thrown at you, laugh at your mistakes. Don't get too embarrassed at every little incident you consider embarrassing. Life is that easy sometimes.

6. Lack of alone time: not finding time for your own self is a gateway to mental stress in the long run.

7. You don't talk to people: chatting on social media is great but they are not real enough conversations as it doesn't truly allow us to understand people thus reducing our experiences and actual feelings which are altogether mentally unhealthy for us.

8. You can't seem to drop that phone for a minute: overusing your phone gives less room for you to rest and regenerate your mind and body. Being addicted to our

phones and staying without it for a while can give off negative effects very similar anxiety or depression if for a longer timeframe.

9. Lack of sleep: sleep enhances emotional and mental capabilities, it helps our bodies rejuvenate. That's why when you lose sleep long enough you may appear as though you've lost your mind.

Here are some natural remedies for mental health:

Mental health treatments could be as natural as ever, from exercises to dieting, to sleep and relaxation but it could also be something more therapeutic in nature like acupuncture, massages and herbal medicines. Acupuncturists believe that mental illnesses such as depression respond well to acupuncture. They also emphasize that acupuncture and massage help cure conditions such as insomnia, anxiety, tense muscles, headaches and pains which happen to millions of people all over the world.

Using natural therapies as those aforementioned directly treats the source of this mental illness even without the use of prescription pills. These natural therapies are cheaper and highly effective as depression and other mental illnesses are reportedly costly to society. In 2005, the cost hit a peak of $10 billion particularly spent on anti-depressant drugs like Prozac and Zoloft.

Acupuncture and massage work in the following ways:

- It triggers the release of endorphins, the body's own internal painkillers
- It both blood circulation and circulation of lymphatic fluids which renews the supply of oxygen to the tissues
- It reduces cortisol (stress hormones)
- It lowers blood pressure, decreases heart rates and relaxes the muscles
- It enhances quick recovery from illnesses
- Acupuncture keeps up the flow of energy that is responsible for physical, emotional and mental wellbeing.
- Acupuncture blocks the sympathetic nerve activity which is triggered by mental stress.

Complementary and Alternative Medicine (CAM) is a program for mental health aimed at self-treatments with a broad range of non-medical substances e.g. Fish oil, exercises, yoga, etc. This is a way to tackle and prevent both physical and mental health problems without drugs or professional supervision.

Cognitive-behavioral therapy

CBT is a therapy that involves using interactions to change a person's thinking and behavior, here deeper levels of communication is seen as a solution to a person's problems. These problems are usually mental and physical health problems. It is common for the treatment of anxiety and depression. CBT emphasizes the fact that your thoughts, feelings physical sensations and actions are purely connected and if your thought and feelings are negative then that negativity will tend to corrupt other parts of the connection. CBT is also used to treat other mental health problems such as bipolar disorder, eating disorders (anorexia and bulimia), borderline personality disorder, panic disorder, phobias, psychosis, post-traumatic stress disorder (PTSD), obsessive-compulsive disorder (OCD), schizophrenia, insomnia, and alcohol abuse. It is also acclaimed to be helpful for the management of long term health conditions like fibromyalgia, irritable bowel syndrome (IBS), chronic fatigue syndrome (CFS).

Sessions with the CBT therapist are to be had once per week or every two weeks, each session lasts for 30 – 60 minutes and about 20 -50 sessions are required in total. CBT can be effective for treating mental health but this may not be suitable for all kinds of mental health problems.

Benefits of CBT

1. It tends to assist where medicine has failed
2. It lasts for a shorter timeframe than other talking therapies
3. It comes in different formats e.g. Groups, help books and apps

Disadvantages of CBT

1. Its success is highly dependent on your devotedness and cooperativeness with your CBT therapist
2. CBT sessions in addition to extra activities can be rather time-consuming
3. It may be initially awkward confronting your emotions and anxieties
4. It may not be suitable for complex mental problems or for people with difficulties in learning

Relationships

Relationships are a good thing only when it is happy. People who find themselves in a toxic relationship would admit to being better off single this is because what they suffer is often more than emotional. A bad relationship can negatively affect your mental, emotional and physical health. If your relationship- leaves you feeling insecure, drained, unhappy, pressurized or bad about yourself, then it's okay to forget about the cute nose and puppy eyes at this point and re-evaluate that relationship. If you are still in doubts and would like to know how directly your physical health is affected by a toxic relationship, then here's how:

That fight or flight mode you often are in makes your body produce excess adrenaline and quickly discards Its excess which can result in fatigue, organ damage and weakened the immune system.

Negative relationships put you at a higher risk of developing heart problems e.g. heart attacks. It also leads to high blood pressure, high blood sugar levels, and obesity. Due to the chemical effects brought about by the constant tension and conflicts in a bad relationship.

In order to ensure a good relationship, there are some helpful basic solutions that can help keep relationship conflicts at bay:

1. Communication – this brings deeper understanding and should be done without raising voices. Good communication also involves being a good listener.
2. Sex – sometimes sex drives of partners are a mismatch even between two people deeply in love. Sometimes it could just be the daily routine in the way of their sex life. Planning towards it in between a tight schedule and trying new ideas can make a big difference.
3. Money – couples fight over money more often than not. Even before weddings, expenses during courtship or wedding could call for serious addressing of money problems. To solve this, partners should be financially transparent and plan their lifestyle according to their finances. There should be transparency over income and debt, financial documents, bank statements, investments, and insurance policies. Also, if one is a saver and the other is a spender,

enjoy the benefits to both as a couple and take a lesson from each other's proclivities. Agree to foot the monthly bills, make budgeting plans and savings together.

4. Home chores division – if both partners work outside the home and likely do not have caretakers, a fair division of labor should be initiated and agreed upon.
5. Make your relationship a privacy
6. Avoid conflicts but if it does arise, calmly address it
7. Trust is the key. Do not distrust your partner. Resolve any hanging issue that is keeping you from trusting each other. Also, be as straightforward as possible in order to earn your partner's trust

The fact is that being 70 and alone is not one of the best situations in the world. In as much as you have every other aspect of your life working for you, you may often feel the need to enjoy the companionship of a life partner, this can help ward off loneliness and other negative feelings it brings. In the long run, relationships are very important as we transit into our autumn years...gracefully.

So, what have we learned?

The next time you come across those exaggerated ads and campaigns on how to grow younger in few days, please skip them like an extra calorie bar on a store shelf having the knowledge that reverse-aging isn't expected to work in days or like the curious case of Benjamin button halfway. Anti-aging, just like aging, is a continuous process that should be a part of your daily living. Yes, we can't stop the clock but we can control our body's response to it. We can keep our mind and body youthful every passing day up till the great beyond.

As the saying goes, when you are beautiful and young it is nature's accident but when you are beautiful and old, it is a work of art and a conscious effort. With the secrets of youth at your fingertips, you will likely look at aging, not as lost youth but a new stage of triumph.

Below are the most useful health websites to keep you abreast of vital health tips and information.

Top 20 best websites for health tips:

1. Netdoctor.co.uk
2. Mayoclinic.com
3. Weightwatcher.com
4. Menshealth.com
5. Womenshealthmag.com
6. www.nih.com
7. Healthline.com

8. www.walgreens.com
9. www.borderlands.com
10. Babycentre.com
11. www.myfitnesspal.com
12. WebMD.com
13. www.medscape.com
14. www.emedicinehealth.com
15. Verywellhealth.com
16. www.facty.com
17. www.fitbit.com
18. www.athenahealth.com
19. www.practo.com
20. Healthinvitro.com

Want more books from Brian Obodeze?

SCAN THE QR CODE
TO SEE OTHER
AWESOME BOOKS FROM THE AUTHOR